From Anesthesia
to X-Rays

From Anesthesia
to X-Rays

INNOVATIONS AND DISCOVERIES
THAT CHANGED MEDICINE FOREVER

Christiane Nockels Fabbri

Foreword by Sandra Panem, PhD

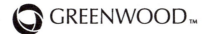

An Imprint of ABC-CLIO, LLC
Santa Barbara, California • Denver, Colorado

Library of Congress Cataloging-in-Publication Data

Names: Nockels Fabbri, Christiane, author. | Panem, Sandra, 1946– writer of foreword.

Title: From anesthesia to X-rays : innovations and discoveries that changed medicine forever / Christiane Nockels Fabbri ; foreword by Sandra Panem.

Description: Santa Barbara, California : ABC-CLIO, LLC, [2017] | Includes bibliographical references and index.

Identifiers: LCCN 2016029285 (print) | LCCN 2016029909 (ebook) | ISBN 9781610695732 (alk. paper) | ISBN 9781610695749 (eISBN) | ISBN 9781610695749 (ebook)

Subjects: | MESH: History of Medicine | Inventions | Diffusion of Innovation

Classification: LCC R702 (print) | LCC R702 (ebook) | NLM WZ 40 | DDC 616.009—dc23

LC record available at https://lccn.loc.gov/2016029285

ISBN: 978-1-61069-573-2
EISBN: 978-1-61069-574-9

21 20 19 18 17   2 3 4 5

This book is also available as an eBook.

Greenwood
An Imprint of ABC-CLIO, LLC

ABC-CLIO, LLC
130 Cremona Drive, P.O. Box 1911
Santa Barbara, California 93116-1911
www.abc-clio.com

This book is printed on acid-free paper ∞

Manufactured in the United States of America

This book is dedicated
To the teachers and students who inspired me, and
To my father, who taught me a critical spirit.

Contents

Foreword

We live in an era where science and technology are rapidly changing all aspects of how we live, work, travel, and communicate. On an almost daily basis we learn of advances in medicine and how as consumers we can take control of our health. Paradoxically, we learn of deadly new diseases, of which Ebola and Zika are two examples. Further, many diseases remain without effective treatment, let alone cures. And although modern medicine leads to an increased life span, there is an alarming increase in the prevalence of diseases that accompany longevity.

How can we make sense of technological and scientific news? Are the findings incremental or revolutionary? Will they change the course of medicine or be forgotten? Christiane Nockels-Fabbri's *From Anesthesia to X-Rays: Innovations and Discoveries That Changed Medicine Forever* provides a welcome framework in which to understand medical innovation.

Written from the perspective of a historian of medicine, Nockels-Fabbri has selected 50 discoveries made from 1796 to 2007 that truly changed the course of medicine. An essay for each describes the discovery; explains how, where, when, and by whom it was made; and most importantly, why it was important. Each entry includes a bibliography and suggested reading list.

The entries are well written, and even the most complex technologies are easily accessible. The holy grail of medical research is to find an effective treatment or cure for a disease. Often the fundamental breakthrough to finding the treatment or cure comes through the understanding enabled by a seemingly unrelated piece of technology. Nockels-Fabbri describes especially well the role of instrumentation in the progress of medical research. For example, the thermometer is a most profound innovation.

In addition to the essays, the book includes a wonderful timeline of medical innovation spanning thousands of years. A series of sidebars provides cultural context for many of the discoveries.

This book can be used in many ways. It is an invaluable resource for students of history, medicine, and science as the beginning inquiry into a particular discovery. For the professional or layperson, it provides an overview of the history of medicine. All readers are likely to return to this book many times.

Sandra Panem, PhD
NeuroNetworksFund
New York, NY
May 2016

Acknowledgments

I am grateful to all—friends, family, colleagues, and patients—who supported my work.

First and foremost, I owe thanks to my husband, Remo Fabbri, for his ongoing encouragement, patient commentary, and incisive insights. He added broad experience and historical background, which helped guide and enrich my research.

I am indebted to my friend and colleague, Mary K. K. Yearl, who gave generous advice and valuable assistance in my early exploration of this project.

Gian D. Fabbri contributed his own much-appreciated time and expertise, and an important entry on a topic near to his heart: Cardiopulmonary Resuscitation, CPR.

I owe a special debt of thanks to my editor, Maxine Taylor, for her guidance and unflagging forbearance; without her, this project would not have come to fruition.

Throughout, my research was supported by the rich resources of the Yale University Library and by its staff, always helpful and willing to go the extra mile.

Introduction

For the student of medicine and history, as for the scientific researcher and medical practitioner, the subject of medical innovation is extremely important. The study of innovations helps explain historical evolution in medicine and the major transformations we have witnessed in population health and life expectancies in recent times. Ongoing developments in immunology, genetics, stem cell research, laboratory tests, and imaging diagnostics challenge traditional understandings of healthcare for patients and practitioners alike. At the same time, as new practices and technologies come into being, they raise important issues for communities and social systems. Here, the role of innovation in limiting healthcare costs while improving outcomes is both critical and controversial.

Yet, the subject of innovation and discovery has been relatively understudied. Reading through this book's short list of medical innovations and discoveries will quickly demonstrate why:

- Innovations and discoveries in medicine or healthcare span a broad range of complex fields and technologies.
- Important discoveries are not always recognized when they occur; their scientific merit or therapeutic significance may take a long time to be validated by experience.
- Innovation aims to solve a problem or results in problem solving often accidentally. This process can at times be entirely serendipitous. Great innovations may solve long-standing problems, or they may open up entire new fields of scientific research.
- By definition, innovation runs counter to tradition and to accepted practice or teaching; it may thus face resistance or even frank opposition from entrenched forces in various parts.

- Successful innovation is often the outcome of competitive research and as such may be fraught with professional disputes or conflicts at times compounded by international rivalries. Therefore, attributing or apportioning just credit can be complicated and may require revision of established historical narratives.

Innovation, defined as the introduction of something new—a new concept, method, or practice—comes from the Latin verb *innovare* ("in"—in, or into—and "novus"—new). Hence, what is new intends to change what is established. Medical innovation changes existing scientific understandings or therapeutic practices. It can also apply to organizational structures or business models aiming to improve healthcare quality, delivery, or access or to reduce healthcare disparities.

Use of the term innovation reflects a pragmatic approach to the study of scientific discovery. Rather than analyzing the theoretical creative, *Eureka*, moment—the sudden exhilaration of discovery—it denotes the process of introduction and implementation into existing medico-social systems. Diffusion or dissemination is the next step, in which innovation is widely adopted. Breakthrough, often synonymous with innovation, is another word used to designate the phenomenon of a publicly recognized major advance in science or technology. However, not all advances are breakthroughs. Cultural historian Bert Hansen, who has traced medical progress and changing popular perceptions of doctors and medicine from the 19th to the 20th century, argues that breakthrough innovation is an advance perceived as substantial, swift, useful, readily practicable, and broadly relevant to many.

Together, these features characterize important innovations as social phenomena that become embedded in popular consciousness. Although innovation can mean different things to different people, in general it is associated with the idea that medical research is capable of providing widespread health benefits.

In popular literature and mass media, the topic of medical innovation has held enduring fascination. Starting with the discoveries of Pasteur and his contemporaries in the 19th century, the fear of sickness, so pervasive in the lives of many, could at last be allayed by the steady march of scientific progress. Ether anesthesia, aseptic surgery, and the germ theory of disease were the first in a series of fundamental advances that effected long-term change in medical practice and fired up popular imagination. They raised new expectations at the same time as they raised the social status of medical practitioners. No longer the quacks or sawbones of early 19th-century "physic," physicians and surgeons were now lionized as valiant figures victorious in the battle against disease. The triumph of laboratory medicine fashioned new heroes and new celebrities. By the mid-1880s Louis Pasteur's name had become a household word in most Western countries.

Over the next few decades, scientific medicine became front-page news, with unprecedented publicity greeting discoveries such as penicillin or the polio vaccine. Already fueled by newspaper and magazine coverage, popular enthusiasm was amplified by book, radio, and film dramatizations. These cultivated public awareness and appreciation for science and encouraged philanthropic and government funding. American children's comic book series such as the 1940s *True Comics*, *Real Heroes*, and *Real Life Comics* further popularized medical history. They starred scientist heroes such as "Death Fighter" Robert Koch and "Famine Fighter" Joseph Goldberger, and they actively explained and promoted medical discoveries. Miracle drugs, lifesaving surgeries, tenacious doctors, and assiduous researchers became symbols of the wonders of modern medicine.

Clearly, medical innovation contributed much to the popularization of science in the early 20th century. But the magic wrought by contemporary breakthroughs together with the spread of mass communication also stimulated a growing public interest in medical history. This in turn prompted science writers to document its narratives. The 1926 classic *Microbe Hunters* by scientist-author Paul de Kruif, a celebrated collection of great medical detective stories, was foremost in sustaining this surge of media attention. *Microbe Hunters* remains in print today and is credited with inspiring "a generation or more of budding young microbiologists." In the same vein, the story of *Dr. Ehrlich's Magic Bullet*, screened in 1940 and chronicling the discovery of salvarsan as a cure for syphilis, was influential in exposing the public to the process of scientific innovation.

Histories of medical innovation were also exploited for commercial use and corporate advertising. "Health Heroes" by the Metropolitan Life Insurance Company and "Famous Doctors" by the Coca-Cola Company are examples of such campaigns. The R. J. Reynolds Company used famous medical pioneers in numerous Camel cigarette ads, where "more doctors smoke Camels than any other cigarette." Listerine, the antiseptic mouthwash named after the founder of sterile surgery Joseph Lister and first formulated in 1879, is still manufactured and sold today.

For historians of medicine, the theme of innovation juxtaposed to tradition becomes part of the study of history as a dynamic process of continuity and change in the evolution of a complex system. Innovation may represent the culmination of the scientific enterprise, located along the way, or at the end, of

In Paris, on November 27, 1895, Swedish innovator Alfred Bernhard Nobel—whose invention of dynamite made him a vast fortune—signed his third and last will. Nobel died a year later, and his will caused a lot of controversy. It was five years before the Nobel Prize could be instituted in accordance with its founder's wishes. The first prize was awarded in 1901.

Excerpt of Alfred Nobel's Last Will and Testament:

I, the undersigned, Alfred Bernhard Nobel, do hereby, after mature deliberation, declare the following to be my last Will and Testament . . . :

[. . .]

The whole of my remaining realizable estate shall be dealt with in the following way: the capital, invested in safe securities by my executors, shall constitute a fund, the interest on which shall be annually distributed in the form of prizes to those who, during the preceding year, shall have conferred **the greatest benefit to mankind**. The said interest shall be divided into five equal parts, which shall be apportioned as follows: **one part to the person who shall have made the most important discovery or invention within the field of physics; one part to the person who shall have made the most important chemical discovery or improvement; one part to the person who shall have made the most important discovery within the domain of physiology or medicine; one part to the person who shall have produced in the field of literature the most outstanding work in an ideal direction; and one part to the person who shall have done the most or the best work for fraternity between nations, for the abolition or reduction of standing armies and for the holding and promotion of peace congresses**. The prizes for physics and chemistry shall be awarded by the Swedish Academy of Sciences; that for physiological or medical work by the Caroline Institute in Stockholm; that for literature by the Academy in Stockholm, and that for champions of peace by a committee of five persons to be elected by the Norwegian Storting. It is my express wish that in awarding the prizes no consideration whatever shall be given to the nationality of the candidates, but that the most worthy shall receive the prize, whether he be a Scandinavian or not.

the researcher's "investigative pathway." This pathway is not, in the words of historian of science Frederic Holmes, a pre-existing route that the investigator *follows*, but one that he or she *creates* while exploring previously uncharted territory. Such studies of innovation have indeed come to replace previous notions of purposeful, teleologic progress in scientific advance, which historians of science had come to regard with suspicion.

Today, biomedical innovation is mostly seen to evolve in a step-wise fashion, taking place in multiple locations with many contributors and increasingly controlled by ethical, legal, economic, and social policies that govern its origination, promotion, and implementation. The medical marketplace itself further complicates attribution of value to innovation. For historians of the field such as John Pickstone, medicine remains a "peculiar market, much influenced by fashion and faith, imponderables, unknowns . . ."

Innovations are not inevitable change. They can be serendipitous, explained in part by social processes or by contextual needs and understandings. Thus, unsanitary conditions together with high mortality rates in mid-19th-century hospitals were instrumental to the undertaking and eventual acceptance of the groundbreaking work of Semmelweis and Lister. Wars, too, were transformative of both practice and power structures. To save lives, military surgeons faced with traumatic injuries and disabilities were forced to innovate. American Civil War surgeons improved amputation techniques and invented the first chloroform inhaler. In the struggle for Italian unification, the 1859 battle of Solferino led to the founding of the Red Cross, bringing about lasting changes in the care of those wounded on battlefields and in future humanitarian efforts on the behalf of those in need. World War I, one of the deadliest conflicts in human history, saw the establishment of the first blood banks. Early orthopedic specialists devised new rehabilitation technologies, including splints and prosthetic limbs, to treat the mutilations and disabilities left behind by the carnage of battle. Many of these innovations had enormous impact on survival rates of the wounded.

Historically, innovations have rarely been subjected to rigorous cost–benefit analysis. We may therefore conclude that the passage of time was efficient enough in filtering value, albeit retrospectively. The vantage point of hindsight in evaluating past innovations does not get to the question of whether these innovations "really worked" within the context of their time and scientific understandings. Nevertheless, many problems were tackled successfully. Anesthesia and antisepsis, for example, even though at the time underlying theoretical foundations had yet to be fully developed, were effective solutions to long-standing problems. Today, in the context of institutional review boards (IRBs) and IRB-controlled research, establishing the value of any given new therapy or technology happens early on in the innovative process, or at any time during or after its adoption. Aside from ethical concerns, a number of other considerations guide the directions of research and decisions regarding implementation. Cost effectiveness and economic motives are ever-increasing issues, especially in capitalist economies. Individual attitudes and beliefs, social networks, corporate priorities, and political and professional interests are some of the other factors at work, as are availability and cost of new drugs or devices.

Ever implicit in the idea of innovation is a value judgment: namely the expectation of improvement or advance over existing, time-honored practices. However, change may not be seen in all quarters as unambiguously good, and further, not all innovations benefit their intended recipients. In 1890, Koch's tuberculin, at first widely acclaimed as a cure for tuberculosis (TB), later stunningly failed even though it eventually found an important application in TB testing. In the 1950s and 1960s, poorly controlled use of thalidomide, one of the most successful prescription drugs in medical history, had disastrous results. Hailed as a wonder drug for insomnia, anxiety, and morning sickness in pregnancy, it caused severe birth defects in thousands of children born to mothers who had taken it. Less clear-cut are the societal and economic consequences of the dismantling of state psychiatric hospitals for the chronic mentally ill in favor of community mental health services. The deinstitutionalization of such patients, although considered more humane by many, has also led to greater incidence of homelessness, victimization, and substance abuse in this population. In the United States, inadequate funding and excessive costs of community psychiatry have frequently resulted in an alternative default mechanism for managing difficult cases: prison incarceration. Ironically, the ensuing explosive growth of private, for-profit prisons underlines the potential risks of breaking with tradition in favor of perceived innovation.

We conclude that innovations do not hold intrinsic or predictable properties, nor do they have uniform outcomes or evolve in linear progression. The effects of newly developed drugs or devices may be provisional, accidental, or even adverse. Patients who experience the measureable—whether intended or inadvertent—consequences of scientific and medical research can, of course, exercise their own, albeit limited, agency. Ultimately, the development and use of medical innovations depend on a combination of factors, all subject to dispute or controversy: economic and political expediency, technological feasibility, and assessment of value in specific individual and social contexts. Importantly, decision and policy-making processes in initiating medical innovation are increasingly central to research direction and support and must, therefore, be as transparent as possible. The goal of innovation, after all, is to best serve the interests of patients, society, and medical science.

In this little book I have aimed to compile a ready-reference encyclopedia that explores key therapeutic, technological, and procedural innovations, as well as discoveries, in the practice of medicine. A major focus is on relatively recent innovations developed over the past 100 years, but fundamental earlier advances in hygiene, public health, and medical technology are also included. My entry selection centers on time-tested, clinical, or therapeutic innovations. Each entry also briefly examines the lasting impact made by these advances.

The topics included were chosen through consultation and discussion with clinical and academic colleagues; through the review of medical literature, as well as consideration of contemporary Nobel Prizes awarded in Physiology or Medicine; and through the lens of my own clinical and academic experience. My little compendium is clearly far from comprehensive. Missing are many innovative technologies and therapies in immunology, oncology, genetics, and other biomedical and surgical fields. These advances are being tried and evolving as we speak, awaiting their own histories and the test of time.

Medicine and healthcare today are undergoing rapid changes, not least because of such burgeoning new technologies, but also as a result of greater interdisciplinary collaboration among diverse fields. Even as medicine is becoming increasingly specialized and, perhaps, hybridized, ever more complex medical information is easily disseminated by powerful new digital representations of body and disease. Increasingly, medicine is "informaticized" even while levels of uncertainty about the clinical relevance of these vast computerized troves of information mount. We are only beginning to understand the challenges raised by our new health technologies, both within the clinic and without. It is my hope that this brief survey of important medical innovations will provide a measure of historical background and context for further exploration and discussion and will stimulate students and the interested general reader to pursue this topic in even greater depth.

Bibliography and Suggested Readings

Eaton, Margaret, and Kennedy, Donald, *Innovation in Medical Technology: Ethical Issues and Challenges*, Baltimore: The Johns Hopkins University Press, 2007.

Garber, Steven, et al., *Challenges to Value-Enhancing Innovation in Health Care Delivery*, Santa Monica: Rand Corporation, 2011.

Hansen, Bert, *Picturing Medical Progress from Pasteur to Polio: A History of Mass Media Images and Popular Attitudes in America*, New Brunswick: Rutgers University Press, 2009.

Pickstone, John, ed., *Medical Innovations in Historical Perspective*, London: MacMillan, 1992.

Reiser, Stanley Joel, *Technological Medicine: The Changing World of Doctors and Patients,* Cambridge: Cambridge University Press, 2009.

Stanton, Jennifer, ed., *Innovations in Health and Medicine: Diffusion and Resistance in the Twentieth Century,* London: Routledge, 2002.

Summers, William C., "Microbe Hunters Revisited," *International Microbiology* 1998, 1: 65–68.

Webster, Andrew, ed., *New Technologies in Health Care: Challenge, Change and Innovation,* Basingstoke: Palgrave MacMillan, 2006.

Procedures and Devices

Angioplasty

What	Medical procedure that aims to open up a blocked blood vessel by means of a flexible tube, or catheter; once in place, the balloon-tipped end of the tube is inflated to widen the obstructed vessel and restore normal blood flow.
Where	United States; Switzerland; Germany
When	1963; 1974
By Whom	Charles Dotter (1920–1985); Andreas Grüntzig (1939–1985)
Importance	Provides effective treatment of vascular disease by minimally invasive percutaneous routes; offers an alternative to open heart surgery for many patients; founded interventional radiology and cardiology.

Angioplasty, from the Greek for "vessel" and "form," is a procedure used to widen narrowed or blocked blood vessels, typically arteries obstructed by atherosclerosis; it is operated through the skin (percutaneous), via the interior opening, or lumen, of the vascular tube (transluminal). Atherosclerotic plaques—deposits of inflammatory cells, cholesterol, and calcium—cause hardening and thickening of arterial walls that can reduce blood flow to the point of blocking it completely. In the peripheral circulation this eventually leads to chronic ulcers, tissue loss, and gangrene. Obstruction of cerebral vessels can lead to strokes or dementia. Coronary obstruction can cause angina and heart attacks.

During angioplasty a thin, flexible, balloon-tipped catheter is introduced into the narrowed vessel and inflated to a predetermined diameter. This compresses the blockage and expands the narrowed vessel, thus improving local blood flow. After inflation the balloon is deflated and withdrawn. A special device called a *stent* (after denture molding material first compounded by 19th-century English dentist Charles Stent, used in World War I to fix skin grafts for the reconstruction of facial wounds) may be inserted to maintain the opening. Angioplasty is based on diagnostic percutaneous catheter techniques introduced in the 1940s and 1950s; it is considered minimally invasive because it is performed on a conscious patient under local anesthesia.

The discovery of angioplasty was serendipitous. In 1963 University of Oregon vascular radiologist Charles Dotter, who a decade earlier had developed one of the first balloon-tipped catheters, inadvertently opened flow in an occluded iliac artery while introducing a catheter during an aortic imaging procedure. He soon envisioned future therapeutic applications, and in 1964 together with his student Melvin Judkins performed an angioplasty on an 82-year-old patient with severe peripheral vascular disease of her left leg. Dotter successfully dilated a narrowed area of the patient's femoral artery, passing a guide wire and then coaxial rigid catheters through the stenosis, and reestablished distal blood flow. The patient promptly recovered, and until her death of heart failure three years later, was, as Dotter reported, "still walking on her own two feet."

Vascular surgeons in the United States did not welcome Dotter's work or forceful attitude. Moreover, his relatively crude technique, used for centuries before to dilate urethral strictures, had limitations: the application of longitudinal shear forces with large rigid tubes to intravascular plaque was risky and awkward. Furthermore, the use of coaxial dilators required progressive enlargement of the percutaneous puncture site. But in Europe, where the treatment of peripheral vascular disease often fell to nonsurgical specialists, Dotter's efforts impelled investigators such as German radiologists Werner Porstmann and Eberhard Zeitler to pursue and refine his methods.

Early attempts to treat arterial obstruction focused on peripheral blood vessels and culminated with the balloon technique pioneered by German physician Andreas Grüntzig, which allowed the percutaneous arterial entry site to be kept to a minimum incision. A critical advance was the addition of a strong inflatable balloon to the tip of a small flexible catheter, making possible dilation via radial rather than shear forces. Grüntzig, who had learned Dotter's method from Zeitler in Germany, first applied it for the recanalization of peripheral and renal arteries. In 1972, he devised an improved Dotter catheter, adding a tougher, sausage-shaped, polyvinyl chloride (PVC) balloon. By 1976 his homemade catheters were being produced by a small U.S. medical instrument manufacturer. They had a double lumen: a distal one for contrast injection and pressure monitoring, and a proximal one for inflating a rigid balloon to a fixed diameter.

In 1977, using a scaled-down double-lumen balloon catheter, Grüntzig and American cardiologist Richard Myler performed the first of several human intraoperative coronary angioplasties at St. Mary's Hospital in San Francisco. The same year, in Zürich, Grüntzig successfully carried out the first coronary angioplasty in a 37-year-old man with severe exertional chest pain due to narrowing of his proximal left anterior descending coronary artery; the patient was awake and stable throughout the procedure. Reporting his case in a 1978 letter to *The Lancet*, Grüntzig correctly predicted that if his technique proved successful in the long term, it would broaden the indications for coronary angiography and provide an alternative treatment for patients with coronary disease. Later that year he published a report of five coronary angioplasties, as well as a first successful balloon dilation of a renal artery stenosis. By 1979 he had dilated more than 50 coronaries with a 64 percent success rate and with no procedural deaths.

Grüntzig's landmark achievement was quickly recognized. It was built on advances not only in coronary angiography but also, by that time, in surgical revascularization; it laid the foundation for interventional cardiology. The medical community embraced the new technique. Over the next few years, improvements in equipment and materials, including refinements in catheters, balloons, and guidewires, allowed its use in increasingly varied clinical settings. At the same time the mechanism of angioplasty at the anatomical level was clarified and helped explain how local tissue disruption could lead to procedural failures and vessel restenosis.

In 1980, Grüntzig moved to Emory University in Atlanta, Georgia. He was 46 in 1985 when he died in a tragic plane crash. Others continued much of the work he had envisioned before his untimely death. New techniques, including atherectomy (excision of arteriosclerotic plaque), stenting, catheter perfusion, and laser angioplasty, extended the original balloon technology and made possible the scouring of atheromas together with preventing acute vascular spasm. In 1986 California cardiologist John Simpson developed a specialized double-lumen catheter with a balloon on one side and a movable cutter on the other to shave off coronary plaque; the U.S. Food and Drug Administration (FDA) approved the device in 1991 for use in coronary disease. Other methods for recanalization include plaque and clot removal through laser technology, high-energy ultrasound, and various hybrid laser–balloon techniques.

In 1987, German physician Ulrich Sigwart reported the first use of intravascular stents. Sigwart's stent configuration was that of a self-expandable spring-like device intended to serve as scaffolding to prevent acute vessel closure or late restenosis and maintain vascular patency. Julio Palmaz at the University of Texas and others developed balloon-expandable metallic mesh stents that eliminated many procedural complications. More recent drug-eluting stents have further improved outcomes. Drug-eluting stents release medication to inhibit local tissue growth and prevent renarrowing of the vessel. All these newer techniques are generally categorized as PCI, or percutaneous coronary intervention; many of them are also applied to peripheral vascular disease.

Angioplasty and related catheter-based interventions have revolutionized the treatment of obstructive atherosclerotic vascular disease. Although not without risk, these innovations have made nonsurgical revascularization an increasingly effective and safe alternative for many patients. Percutaneous transluminal angioplasty (PTA), with and without stenting, has become standard practice in all limb arteries, as well as in other parts of the body, including the coronary and carotid arteries. Coronary angioplasty has become one of the most common medical interventions in the world and is increasingly performed as a same-day procedure. In the United States, the number of PTAs to treat coronary disease now exceeds that of surgical bypass grafts.

Bibliography and Suggested Readings

Baim, Donald S., ed., *Grossman's Cardiac Catheterization, Angiography, and Intervention*, 7th ed., Philadelphia: Lippincott, Williams & Wilkins, 2006.

King, Spencer B., "Angioplasty from Bench to Bedside to Bench," *Circulation* 1996; 93(9): 1621–1629.

King, Spencer B., "The Development of Interventional Cardiology," *Journal of the American College of Cardiology* March 1998, 31(4s2): 64B–88B.

Mauro, Matthew A., et al., *Image-Guided Interventions*, 2nd ed., Philadelphia: Saunders/Elsevier, 2014.

Morell, Michael S., *Essential Interventional Cardiology*, 2nd ed., Philadelphia: Saunders/Elsevier, 2008.

Mueller, Richard L., and Sanborn, Timothy A., "The History of Interventional Cardiology: Cardiac Catheterization, Angioplasty, and Related Interventions," *American Heart Journal* 1995; 129(1): 146–172.

Payne, Misty M., "Charles Theodore Dotter: The Father of Intervention," *Texas Heart Institute Journal* 2001, 28(1): 28–38.

Roguin, Ariel, "Stent: The Man and Word Behind the Coronary Metal Prosthesis," *Circulation: Cardiovascular Interventions* 2011, 4: 206–209.

von Schmilowski Eva, and Swanton, R. H., *Essential Angioplasty*. Somerset: John Wiley & Sons, 2011.

Blood Transfusion

What	Intravenous transfer of blood or blood components from the circulation system of one individual into that of another.
Where	England; France; United States
When	1665; 1667; 1818; 1907; 1915
By Whom	Richard Lower (1631–1691); Jean-Baptiste Denys (1643–1704); James Blundell (1790–1877); Reuben Ottenberg (1882–1959); Richard Lewisohn (1875–1961)

Importance   Dramatic lifesaving measure in cases of severe hemorrhage, providing a way to replace lost blood; allows prevention of cardiovascular shock in surgery and trauma; makes possible treatment of chronic blood disorders.

Transferring blood from one individual to another is a recent practice, but the concept of transfusion has an old history. Blood was long understood to be the body's vital force, essential to life; its loss was associated with weakness and death. Many cultures believed in the power of blood, and to this day it is consumed in various forms, often for medicinal purposes. The scientific use of blood as a therapeutic product can be traced back to the 17th century, when early experiments with direct transfusion were likely inspired by William Harvey's 1628 description of blood circulating within a closed system. The greatest advances in transfusion medicine, however, were stimulated by the global conflicts of the first half of the 20th century. During World War II blood transfusion became a practical reality, and in modern medicine it is one of the most important lifesaving interventions.

An early pioneer in studying the effects of blood transfer from one animal to another was Oxford physician Richard Lower. He performed a series of dog-to-dog transfusions that were documented by the Royal Society in May 1665. It was not long before Lower and others investigated animal-to-human transfusions. Among them was Jean-Baptiste Denys, physician to Louis XIV of France. Denys is credited with having performed the first xenotransfusion (transfer of blood between species) when in 1667 he transfused the blood of a lamb into a teenage boy suffering from a chronic fever, apparently without ill effects. A few months later Lower performed a similar experiment, chronicled by London diarist Samuel Pepys: the transfusion of sheep's blood into a former minister who suffered from mental illness.

Denys, who investigated the potential of transfusion not only to replace blood loss but also to treat disease, preferred the use of animal blood for his experiments for he thought it less likely "to be rendered impure by passion or vice." Indeed, blood was generally believed to carry a person's—or an animal's—physical and mental qualities and characteristics, and could convey these to the recipient. The blood of a lamb was favored for transfusion because this animal was known for its mild temperament.

The practice of transfusion had elicited strong disapproval from the medical establishment in both France and England. Many conservative physicians refused to accept Harvey's theory of blood circulation and were opposed to transfusion. Besides, traditional medical therapies involved removing blood from the patient by bloodletting or leeching, not supplying it from a foreign body. Denys's final experiments had moreover resulted in fatal outcomes, likely due to what we now recognize as hemolytic transfusion reactions. The French parliament outlawed transfusions in 1678. The Royal Society in London also withdrew its support, and Pope Innocent XI in 1679 issued a decree prohibiting Catholics from participating in blood transfusions.

After this backlash, the practice fell into disrepute until the early 1800s when noted British obstetrician James Blundell revived interest in the scientific basis of transfusion. Blundell, "appalled at [his] own helplessness at combating fatal hemorrhage during delivery," initially experimented with transfusions between dogs, but soon followed the teaching of his Edinburgh colleague John Henry Leacock that donor and recipient must be of the same species. In 1818 he performed the first human-to-human blood transfusion upon a man suffering from gastric cancer. Although the patient died, Blundell persisted in his research and in 1829 successfully treated a woman for severe postpartum hemorrhage with blood transfused from his assistant.

Blundell had noted that direct vein-to-vein transfusion was not practical due to clotting, whereas connecting a donor's vein to a recipient's artery by a fine tube was more effective. He also developed an indirect technique using a syringe for drawing blood from the donor and immediately injecting it into the recipient's vein. He described this process in several papers, noting the importance of removing air from the instrument prior to use, as well as the need for swiftness to avoid the problems of blood clotting.

Clotting, or coagulation of blood, could block tubing or other apparatus and was a major problem that stood in the way of successful human-to-human transfusion in the 19th century. Increasingly, blood from which the platelet clot (fibrin) had been removed was used. A variety of methods were employed to accomplish this, most of them involving stirring and straining of the blood. Later, sodium bicarbonate was added as an anticoagulant. It would take another 50 years before the development of effective anticoagulation methods. There was also debate about the benefits of using blood rather than saline solution. American surgeon George Washington Crile found that in surgical shock, blood was more effective in maintaining blood pressure, and in his subsequent investigations continued the search for better and safer transfusion methods. Here he drew on technical innovations in the suturing of blood vessels, especially the end-to-end anastomosis of arteries and veins developed by French surgeon Alexis Carrel.

Much other work done in the later 19th century was to refine surgical techniques and transfusion apparatus. Blood groups had not yet been discovered, which meant that little was understood about when donor blood would be compatible with that of the recipient. The severe reactions that often and unpredictably followed many transfusions were mostly attributed to the introduction of air bubbles into the patient's circulation. Transfusion remained a controversial, dangerous, and invasive procedure, only to be used as a last resort. It was not until Karl Landsteiner's discovery of the human ABO blood groups in 1900 that the phenomenon of blood group incompatibility was explained. Landsteiner demonstrated that the serum of some people agglutinated, or clumped, the red cells of others due to different antigens and antibodies. This immunologic reaction was what led to intravascular hemolysis, the breaking up of red cells, which could be fatal.

Landsteiner had suggested his findings might be applicable to blood transfusion practice, and in 1907 American physician Reuben Ottenberg performed the first transfusion after typing and crossmatching donor and recipient blood to ensure compatibility. Nevertheless, it took until the end of World War I for preliminary "cross-agglutination" screening to become routine in clinical practice. In 1914 and 1915 Belgian Adolph Hustin, Argentinian Luis Agote, and American Richard Lewisohn found that adding sodium citrate to fresh blood delayed clotting. This allowed for longer storage and eliminated the technical difficulties of direct transfusion. A later glucose additive improved red cell preservation. Transfusion was now therapeutically viable.

The first voluntary blood donor program was organized in London in 1921. The advent of blood banking in the 1930s—made possible by the recently developed

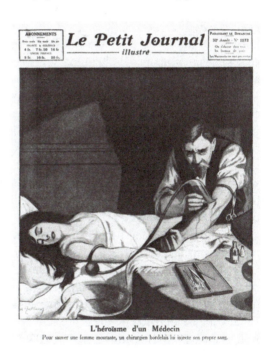

L'héroïsme d'un Médecin
Pour sauver une femme mourante, un chirurgien bordelais lui injecte son propre sang.

Until the advent of blood typing and banking, direct transfusion was a last resort in cases of severe hemorrhage. A popular French weekly in 1921 illustrated a surgeon's desperate attempt to transfuse a dying patient with his own blood. The same year, the British Red Cross organized the first voluntary blood donor program. (U.S. National Library of Medicine/NIH) electrical refrigeration—was a major innovation, allowing the use of preserved rather than fresh blood. In 1939 the new British Army Blood Transfusion Service started the Army Blood Supply Depot (ABSD), the first military transfusion service in the world. In 1941, the first Red Cross blood donor center opened in New York City. Surgeon Charles Drew, medical director of the *Blood for Britain Program*, developed criteria for mass collection, which ultimately yielded over 10 million pints of blood; most of this was shipped to the European and Pacific fronts. Douglas Kendrick, who directed the U.S. Army blood program, later wrote that mortality rates in combat were reduced by 50 percent because of the availability of "prompt and adequate resuscitation, in which whole blood and plasma play major roles."

Methods for collecting, processing, and storing blood supplies became increasingly sophisticated. Techniques to preserve dried blood products, developed in the late 1930s, were followed by the introduction of freeze-drying processes for human plasma. By 1960, mass-produced plastic sets for blood collection and transfusion allowed for aseptic separation and storage of blood components.

Together with blood typing and crossmatching, the development of practical anticoagulation and storage methods established transfusion as a critical lifesaving intervention in 20th-century medicine. Today, the replacement of blood lost in childbirth, surgery, or trauma has become routine and overwhelmingly safe. The major indication for transfusion remains severe hemorrhage, where transfused blood restores both volume and oxygenation of tissues. Transfusion is also important in treating other conditions, including hemophilia and certain types of anemia.

Yet, even now, blood transfusion is not without risk. Early 20th century reports confirmed transmission of diseases such as measles, malaria, and syphilis, making the need for microbial screening of blood donations increasingly clear. Today, diagnostic systems that ensure all donated blood is screened for transmissible infections are central to every national blood program. In the United States, all blood products are screened for bacterial contamination, as well as for syphilis, hepatitis B and C, HIV, human T-cell lymphotropic virus (HTLV) and West Nile virus; cytomegalovirus (CMV) and Chagas antibody testing are often included. Still, globally, significant variations exist in overall quality and effectiveness of blood-screening processes. As a result, in many countries transfusion recipients remain at unacceptable risk of acquiring preventable infections.

Bibliography and Suggested Readings

Centers for Disease Control and Prevention, "Blood Safety Basics," 2013, http://www.cdc.gov/bloodsafety/basics.html.

Harding, Anthony J., "A Brief History of Blood Transfusion," 2005, https://www.ibms
.org/go/nm:history-blood-transfusion

Learoyd, Philip, "The History of Blood Transfusion Prior to the 20th Century," *Transfusion Medicine* 2012, 22: 308–314; 372–376.

Lederer, Susan E., *Flesh and Blood: Organ Transplantation and Blood Transfusion in 20th Century America,* Oxford: Oxford University Press: 2008.

Roux, Françoise A., Saï, Pierre, and Deschamps, Jack-Yves, "Xenotransfusions, Past and Present," *Xenotransplantation* 2007, 14: 208–216.

Cardiopulmonary Resuscitation (CPR)

What	A life-sustaining technique in which rescuer(s) provide artificial respiration and rhythmic chest compressions to oxygenate and circulate blood through the bodies of persons with cardiac arrest or life-threatening arrhythmias.
Where	Baltimore, Maryland
When	1960
By Whom	Peter Safar (1924–2003); James Elam (1918–1995); William Kouwenhoven (1886–1975); Guy Knickerbocker (1932–); James Jude (1928–2015)
Importance	Major advance in resuscitation technique, associated with significant increases in patient survival after cardiovascular events; brought the ability to save lives out of the hospital and into the hands of the general population through a standardized, easy-to-learn, nonsurgical technique that could be performed without specialized equipment.

On April 21, 2012, 14-year-old Evan Blackstone had just finished an off-season workout with his team when his heart stopped beating and he fell to the ground. Had Evan collapsed prior to 1960, he might have received a flogging, been draped over a trotting horse, or even had smoke pumped into his rectum with a bellows. Whether he would have survived is anyone's guess, but instead, Evan's coaches immediately began cardiopulmonary resuscitation (CPR) and Evan survived. Later, surgeons would go on to repair the congenital heart defect that lead to Evan's cardiac arrest, but credited the coaches' swift action with saving Evan's life.

Today, CPR has become a familiar lifesaving technique around the world and has transformed bystanders into potential lifesavers. The breakthrough integration of rescue breathing and chest compressions did not occur until 1960, but the roots of modern CPR date back thousands of years. Literary references to resuscitation of the dead date to 800 B.C., when the Bible described Elisha reviving a boy by putting his mouth upon the child's mouth and causing the flesh to warm (2 Kings 4:34). Chinese physician Zhang Zhongjing described artificial respiration in his *Treatise on Febrile Diseases Caused by Cold*, which includes accounts of a lifesaving technique remarkably similar to modern Western CPR:

> One person should put his feet against the shoulders of the victim and pull on his hair, rendering it taut [opening the airway]. One person should put his hands on the victim's chest and compress rhythmically.

In ancient Western medicine, resuscitation attempts focused primarily on warming or stimulating the body to counteract cooling of the corpse or to rouse the deceased. Caregivers would apply hot water or ashes or whip the dead to stimulate a response. In the 16th century practice turned to artificial respiration. The anatomist Vesalius is credited with the first mechanical ventilation via tracheostomy. Later, fireplace bellows were used to inflate the lungs, but this practice fell out of favor following the 1827 demonstration of French surgeon Leroy d'Étiolles that overfilling of the lungs itself could cause death. Earlier, the Paris Academy of Sciences had recommended mouth-to-mouth resuscitation; this technique was soon abandoned due to skepticism about the value of "devitalized" air.

In 1767 and 1774, the newly founded Dutch Society for the Recovery of Drowned Persons and the British Royal Humane Society formalized resuscitation methods for victims of drowning. Their efforts contributed to disseminating these techniques outside of traditional hospital environments. Practices focused on warming the victim, stimulating him using strong odors or rectal fumigation, and assisting respiration using a bellows after clearing the lungs of water. Rhythmic ventilation was further attempted as rescuers tried rolling victims back and forth over barrels, draping them over trotting horses, or rolling them from side to side to force air into and out of the lungs. Among these methods, the latter gained the endorsement of the Royal Humane Society and was widely adopted. Its developer, Marshall Hall, demonstrated that his technique could produce respiratory volumes approaching those of healthy adults.

Pulmonary resuscitation had always been the main focus of lifesaving techniques, but the advent of modern anesthesia in the mid-1800s saw an increase in intraoperative cardiac arrests as a result of the low therapeutic index of chloroform. This led physicians to explore ways of restarting the heart following cardiac arrest. In 1891, surgeon Friedrich Maass performed the first successful external cardiac massage as a last-ditch effort to save a young boy whose heart had stopped while undergoing surgery. He applied direct compression to the cardiac region, working fast and vigorously; after an hour of effort, he detected a pulse, and the child was able to breathe without assistance. Yet Maass's technique was not widely adopted; it would not be "rediscovered" until the 1960s. Instead, open-chest cardiac massage gained preeminence following a first such resuscitation by Norwegian surgeon Kristian Igelsrud in 1901. By 1952 success rates for internal cardiac massage approached 33 percent. Still, this method required a surgical facility and trained practitioners and was of little use in providing early rescue to victims in the field where most cardiac arrests occur.

In 1958, Johns Hopkins graduate student Guy Knickerbocker rediscovered the effectiveness of closed-chest compressions. Knickerbocker was researching defibrillation in William Kouwenhoven's electrophysiology lab, when his laboratory dog suddenly developed ventricular fibrillation. He began rhythmic thoracic compressions, recalling the spikes in blood pressure he had observed when applying heavy paddles to animals' chests. He continued compressions for about 20 minutes until an electrical defibrillator could be located to revive the dog fully. On this chance discovery Kouwenhoven and collaborator James Jude subsequently built a body of research. They published their findings in 1960, reporting a 70 percent survival rate in 20 patients receiving closed-chest compressions, thus laying the foundation for modern CPR. Their closed-chest technique now made it possible for lay people, outside of the hospital, to treat cardiac arrest.

Skepticism regarding the efficacy of breathing used, exhaled air into a patient's lungs had persisted until 1954, when U.S. physician James Elam proved that this air was rich enough in oxygen to sustain life. Together with anesthesiologist Peter Safar, who devised the "head-tilt, chin-lift," and "jaw-thrust" techniques for maintaining an open airway, Elam developed standards for mouth-to-mouth rescue breathing, which were adopted by the U.S. military in 1957 and widely disseminated among servicemen. In 1961, Safar, taking a cue from the Baltimore Fire Department where rescue squads had trained independently in his own rescue breathing and Kouwenhoven's chest compressions, integrated the two groups' pioneering techniques. Today, guidelines and best practices continue to evolve, but Safar's "ABCs (Airway, Breathing, and Circulation) of Resuscitation," laid the groundwork for modern CPR.

Physicians early on realized the lifesaving potential that such a simple technique could have, particularly because most cardiac arrests take place at home. Notwithstanding the National Academy of Sciences's warnings against educating the general population in CPR, surgeon Claude Beck soon began teaching laypeople in Cleveland. In 1970, a Seattle group led by cardiologist Leonard Cobb trained over 100,000 laypersons, developed a rapid-response system, and instructed 911 operators in how to coach bystanders in CPR. In 1974, the American Heart Association (AHA) and the National Academy of Sciences reversed their position and endorsed widespread lay training, effectively giving their blessing to massive public education efforts by such organizations as the AHA and American Red Cross.

The widespread adoption of CPR has allowed countless victims to survive long enough to receive more advanced life support. Bystander CPR establishes a critical first step in treating cardiac arrest in the field, where prompt intervention makes a significant difference in ultimate survival. Though field-administered CPR in isolation is associated with a relatively low 10 percent survival rate, subsequent defibrillation increases survival twofold to threefold. With over 300,000 sudden cardiac arrests in North America annually, CPR is crucial; as best practices are refined and reach even greater portions of the population, its impact will continue to grow.

Bibliography and Suggested Readings

Carveth, Stephan, "Standards for Cardiopulmonary Resuscitation and Emergency Cardiac Care," *JAMA* 1974, 227(7): 796–797.

Cooper, J. A., "Cardiopulmonary Resuscitation: History, Current Practice, and Future Direction," *Circulation* 2006, 114: 2839–2849.

Deng, Y., *Introduction to Chinese Culture: Ancient Chinese Inventions.* Cambridge: Cambridge University Press, 2011.

Flynn, R., "A Dying Dog, a Slow Elevator, and 50 Years of CPR," *Hopkins Medicine Magazine* Winter 2011, 28–35.

Gordon, A. S., "Cardiopulmonary Resuscitation Conference Proceedings," in *National Research Council (U.S.). Ad Hoc Committee on Cardiopulmonary Resuscitation, Washington:* National Academies, 1967.

Hurt, R., "Modern Cardiopulmonary Resuscitation—Not So New After All," *Journal of the Royal Society of Medicine* 2005, 98: 327–331.

O'Connor, W. J., *Founders of British Physiology: A Biographical Dictionary, 1820–1885.* Manchester: Manchester University Press, 1988.

Sisco, A., *"CPR Saves Young Athlete's Life at Lusher Charter School in New Orleans,"* 2012, http://blog.nola.com/new_orleans/2012/05/cpr_saves_young_athletes_life.html.

Wang, Z., and Xie, P. *History and Development of Chinese Medicine.* Amsterdam: IOS Press, 1999.

Zhang, A. A., "*A Brief History of Time: CPR (Cardiopulmonary Resuscitation),*" 2008, http://cockroachcatcher.blogspot.com/2008/08/brief-history-of-time-cpr.html.

Cataract Surgery

What	Surgical extraction and replacement of ocular lens with artificial implant.
Where	London; New York
When	1949; 1967
By Whom	Harold Ridley (1906–2001); Charles Kelman (1930–2004)
Importance	Restores vision and significantly improves quality of life; one of the most common and safest surgical procedures performed in older adults.

Cataracts are the most frequent cause of visual loss in later life. Caused by progressive clouding and hardening of the eye's crystalline lens, the condition can lead to severe visual impairment, if not total blindness. In ancient Rome, cataracts (from the Latin "waterfall") were thought to be due to thickened humors that had seeped into the eye from the brain. Cataract surgery was documented as early as the fifth century B.C.; early procedures are described in Sanskrit, Arabic, and medieval texts. The traditional operation, called "couching" of cataracts, involved dislocating the opacified lens from its fibrous anchors (zonules) and pushing it into the eye's vitreous cavity, out of the line of sight. This procedure could only be performed when the lens had become hard and rigid enough to allow the operator to insert a fine sharp instrument and break the lens's zonular attachments in order to displace it. The process would restore vision but not visual focus or capacity for accommodation.

Eye surgery was among the earliest of the modern surgical specialties to develop. Extractions of the lens were first reported in the 1750s but they were technically difficult and had potential for serious complications. Most practitioners, including barber surgeons and itinerant oculists, continued to use the old couching technique until well into the 19th century. By the late 1800s complete removal of the lens within its capsular sac had replaced the old couching method. Such extractions were made safer as well as more effective and practicable by the advent of sterile techniques and the use of topical anesthesia, introduced in 1884 by Vienna ophthalmologist Carl Koller.

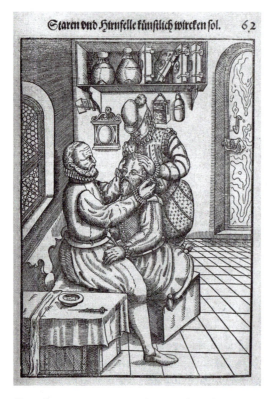

Staren vnd Hirnfelle künstlich wircken sol.   62

Couching a cataract, as depicted in the 1583 *Ophthalmoduleia* by Dresden surgeon Georg Bartisch. This first German textbook of ophthalmology contained 91 woodcut illustrations—some using ingenious movable flaps enabling the reader to "dissect" the eye. A detailed discussion of treatments and surgical techniques accompanied the images. Bartisch was court oculist to the Duke of Saxony and known for skillful cataract operations, for which he recommended using gold-plated needles. (History of Science Collections/University of Oklahoma Libraries)

This type of lens removal, known as intracapsular cataract extraction, or ICCE, was standard until World War II and involved removing the entire opaque lens within its capsule by means of a large incision around the cornea. Surgery was restricted to so-called "mature" cataracts, those hard enough not to break up during surgery because fragments that fell into the vitreous space could cause inflammation. While the wound healed, patients were kept immobilized with sandbags around their head and occlusive dressings covering their eyes. Successful operations would allow light to pass unimpeded to the retina; however, it could not be focused into a clear image. Thick, "pebble" or "Coke-bottle" glasses could provide only a small measure of postoperative correction. Moreover, in the elderly, prolonged bed rest and eye occlusion often led to infection, urinary tract obstruction, clots and pulmonary emboli, or even delirium. For most patients, therefore, the risk of such perioperative complications made the intervention a measure of last resort.

A first major advance was the introduction of techniques for removing the lens but leaving the intact posterior capsule in place; this prevented lens material from falling into the vitreous cavity. Called extracapsular extraction (ECCE), the technique allowed less advanced cataracts to be removed because residual fragments could be aspirated without loss of vitreous humor. Size of the incision was also reduced, and use of fine suture material resulted in better outcomes.

The major problem that remained was the optical correction of aphakia (the absence of a lens). In the 1940s British ophthalmologist Harold Ridley had started experimenting with a new ECCE technique in which the extracted portion of the lens would be replaced. The problem was not only to insert a new lens, but also to find an adequate substitute material. Plastic contact lenses, invented in the 1930s, seemed to be tolerated. Experience with wounded fighter pilots had demonstrated that intraocular shrapnel from shattered windshields did not always lead to significant eye damage. Ridley enlisted the help of a chemical engineer and an ophthalmic product manufacturer to produce a clear, inert, lightweight, "clinical quality" Plexiglas material, which they called *Perspex CQ*. Together, they created the first artificial lens, designed for insertion in the posterior chamber of the eye. Using this approach, in 1949 Ridley successfully implanted the first intraocular lens (IOL) into the eye of a 45-year-old woman whose cataract he had removed some three months earlier.

Ridley's early implants had a number of defects. Lenses were relatively thick and heavy; handmade, they were poorly standardized, and there were no effective ways to sterilize them. Postoperative inflammation or dislocation was common, and initial failure rates forcing implant removal were as high as 15 percent. However, Ridley's technique produced a better visual field and an optically normal eye.

Subsequent innovators experimented with anterior chamber implants, but this caused corneal edema, and even glaucoma, and was eventually abandoned. The critical development that transformed Ridley's ECCE method into a now-routine surgical procedure was the introduction in 1967 of phacoemulsification surgery by New York ophthalmologist Charles Kelman. Kelman's technique—literally a liquefying or pulverizing of the lens and reportedly inspired by his dentist's ultrasonic probe—used high-frequency ultrasound vibration to break the cataract into minute fragments that could then be aspirated, leaving the posterior lens capsule intact. A handheld instrument consisting of an ultrasonic vibrating needle and a probe for irrigation and aspiration of debris permitted the operator to perform the procedure through a tiny incision. Afterward, an intraocular lens (IOL) implant would be inserted. Nowadays, newer foldable implants have replaced the conventional rigid lenses. They can be introduced to unfold within the remaining lens capsule so that incisions do not have to be enlarged.

Phacoemulsification revolutionized cataract surgery and led to its becoming a safe, standardized ambulatory procedure that can usually be performed in a few hours. By the end of the 20th century, cataract surgery and IOL replacement had become one of the safest, most common outpatient operations. Currently, IOL implants also restore good distance vision. Lenses that will accommodate, eliminating the need for reading glasses, will likely be available in the future.

Bibliography and Suggested Readings

Apple, David, *Sir Harold Ridley and His Fight for Sight: He Changed the World so That We May Better See It*, Thorofare: Slack, 2006.

Bellan, Lorne, "The Evolution of Cataract Surgery: The Most Common Eye Procedure in Older Adults," *Geriatrics and Aging* 2008, 11(6): 328–332.

Kwitko, Marvin L., and Kelman, Charles D., eds., *History of Modern Cataract Surgery*, The Hague: Kugler Publications, 1998.

Webster, Andrew, ed., *New Technologies in Health Care: Challenge, Change and Innovation*, New York: Palgrave MacMillan, 2006.

Dialysis

What	Blood filtering process used in patients with acute or chronic renal failure; removes metabolic waste products and excess fluid normally excreted by the kidney through an external filter, or dialyzer.
Where	Canada; Germany; Holland; Sweden; United States
When	1924; 1943
By Whom	Nils Alwall (1906–1986); Georg Haas (1886–1971); Willem Kolff (1911–2009); Gordon Murray (1884–1972); Beldon Scribner (1921–2003)
Importance	Revolutionized the treatment of kidney disease, making possible the survival of millions of affected patients; provided the impetus for the development of artificial organs and technological medicine.

One of the most important functions of the kidney is the excretion of soluble metabolic waste products in the urine. When this process fails, the accumulation of excess fluid, electrolytes, and toxic metabolites results in progressive fatigue, nausea, weakness, confusion, and ultimately vomiting, coma, and death. Dialysis, also called renal dialysis or hemodialysis, is the process of purifying the blood of patients with kidney failure and then returning it to the patient's bloodstream.

The hemodialyzer is a machine capable not only of removing accumulated toxic substances but also of supplying necessary sugars, salts, and amino acids, thus replacing an important part of normal kidney function. During dialysis, two liquids, the patient's blood on one side and a sterile dialysate solution on the other, are separated by a semipermeable membrane and exchange small dissolved particles by diffusion. Large particles such as red and white blood cells, platelets, and proteins cannot penetrate the membrane. Needed diffusible substances are added to the sterile solution to offset losses or deficiencies. Ultrafiltration, during which water along with solutes is forced through the dialyzer membrane by a positive pressure differential, prevents excess water from diluting the blood.

Effective treatment for renal failure began only in the mid-20th century, with Dutch physician Willem Kolff's first hemodialysis machine. Kolff's innovation, as many others, was the product of accumulated scientific knowledge and expertise, as well as individual ingenuity. At the time, the pathophysiological mechanism of kidney failure was well understood, but in the absence of viable therapies most physicians accepted as inevitable the fatal outcome of end-stage kidney disease. Urea, one of the main waste products of protein metabolism known to accumulate in renal failure, had been identified in the 19th century. The chemical process of osmosis—the movement of water and solutes across a porous membrane according to their respective concentration gradients—was elucidated around the same time. Scottish chemist Thomas Graham in 1854 had first described dialysis as a method of separating highly diffusible substances, or crystalloids, from slowly diffusing colloids.

Early attempts at kidney dialysis were unsuccessful. Among the many technical difficulties preventing mechanical extracorporeal blood filtering were lack of effective anticoagulants, as well as clinically usable semipermeable membranes. German physician Georg Haas in 1924 performed the first human hemodialysis using the leech extract hirudin as an anticoagulant together with collodion membranes. However, these materials were fragile and toxic; neither proved practical for clinical use, and Haas abandoned his research a few years later.

In 1937, the naturally occurring anticlotting agent heparin still used today became available in a standardized purified form. The same year, New York hematologist William Thalhimer in his work on exchange transfusion used heparin with cellophane as an experimental dialysis membrane. Cellophane, a thin film of cellulose widely employed for sausage tubing, was sturdy and durable, inexpensive, easily sterilized, and proved to have excellent diffusion characteristics.

The ready availability of pure heparin together with cellophane membranes and tubing set the stage for the development of effective human dialysis. Three researchers working independently in the early 1940s are credited with this pioneering advance: Willem Kolff of the Netherlands, Nils Alwall of Sweden, and Gordon Murray of Canada. Kolff's role is generally seen as primary. He was the first to succeed in carrying out the procedure and obtaining beneficial results. Moreover, he was an energetic advocate of therapeutic dialysis and freely distributed prototypes of his new artificial kidney machine. By his own report, the idea of removing urea and other metabolic retention products from the blood of uremic patients grew in him when in 1938 he was faced with a young man slowly dying of renal failure due to chronic nephritis. He thought then that if he could find a way to eliminate the toxic waste products that build up in such patients, he might keep them alive until their kidneys rebounded.

Kolff correctly assumed that blood urea, which could be measured, was a marker for the accumulation of toxic metabolites. He carried out *in vitro* experiments to calculate the appropriate surface area of the dialysis membrane, duration of the exchange, and adequate replacement of essential electrolytes. In the midst of the German occupation of the Netherlands, he developed a rotating drum dialysis machine and proved extraordinarily resourceful in constructing his artificial kidney with scarce available materials and secret support from local manufacturers. Kolff performed the first human dialysis in September 1943; it would take another 15 patients and two more years before he could claim success. This was in late 1945 when he saved the life of his 17th dialysis patient, a 67-year-old woman suffering from acute renal failure; she lived another seven years.

A 2009 *New York Times* obituary described Kolff's device as "an exemplar of Rube Goldberg ingenuity. It consisted of 50 yards of sausage casing wrapped around a wooden drum set into a salt solution. The patient's blood was drawn from a wrist artery and fed into the casings. The drum was rotated, removing impurities. To get the blood safely back into the patient, Dr. Kolff copied the design of a water-pump coupling used in Ford motor engines. Later he used orange juice cans and a clothes washing machine to build his apparatuses."

Further advances in the design of the dialyzer apparatus were made in the late 1940s and 1950s. Nils Alwall built a system using a vertical stationary drum and circulating dialysate and applied hydrostatic pressure to achieve ultrafiltration. Kolff and others made additional improvements.

Kolff's invention was a direct challenge to established medical theory and practice. Its acceptance was slow, except in the United States where John Merrill at Boston's Brigham Hospital refined Kolff's original design. The Kolff-Brigham machine was successfully used during the Korean War where it dramatically decreased mortality in the acutely injured. The military's clear-cut results paved the way for wider acceptance. Starting in the mid-1950s, the artificial kidney, together with specialized dialysis units, gradually became part of the routine treatment of acute kidney failure.

A crucial development came in 1960 when Seattle nephrologist Belding Scribner introduced a silastic device fitted with Teflon tips to function as an arteriovenous shunt. This allowed not only for continuous circulation when the patient was not connected to the machine, but also eliminated clotting and—importantly—provided ready vascular access for repeated dialyses. The Scribner shunt ushered in a new phase in clinical hemodialysis, for it opened the door to regular long-term therapy for patients with chronic end-stage renal disease (ESRD). Like Kolff, Scribner was an influential advocate for dialysis; his efforts contributed to the passage of the 1972 U.S. Medicare amendment providing extensive coverage for dialysis services. Nowadays, thousands of ESRD patients undergo dialysis several times a week and are often being kept alive until kidney transplantation is possible.

Willem Kolff's dialysis machine was the first to replace the function of an organ. His artificial kidney not only saved countless lives, but also ushered in an era of technological medicine in which biomedical engineers increasingly entered the medical marketplace to construct fresh, manmade body parts.

Dr. Kolff, often described as the father of artificial organs, immigrated to the United States in 1950; a few years later he developed a membrane oxygenator for use in bypass surgery, as well as a first artificial heart. According to the *New York Times*, he "continued to work on artificial organs . . . until he retired in 1997 at the age of 86, maintaining the same philosophy he had held to when developing the artificial heart. 'If a man can grow a heart,' Dr. Kolff always insisted, 'he can build one.' "

Bibliography and Suggested Readings

Blakeslee, Sandra, "Willem Kolff, Doctor Who Invented Kidney and Heart Machines, Dies at 97," 2009, http://www.nytimes.com/2009/02/13/health/13kolff.html?page wanted=all&_r=0

Cameron, J. Stewart, "Practical Haemodialysis Began with Cellophane and Heparin: The Crucial Role of William Thalhimer *(1884–1961),*" *Nephrology Dialysis Transplantation* 2000, 15(7): 1086–1091.

Kolff, Willem J., "First Clinical Experience with the Artificial Kidney," *Annals of Internal Medicine* 1965, 62: 608–619.

Noordwijk, Jacob, *Dialysing for Life: The Development of the Artificial Kidney,* Dordrecht: Springer, 2001.

Peitzman, Steven J., *Dropsy, Dialysis, Transplant: A Short History of Failing Kidneys.* Baltimore: Johns Hopkins University Press, 2008.

Quinton, Wayne, Dillard David, and Scribner, Belding H., "Cannulation of Blood Vessels for Prolonged Hemodialysis," *Transactions—American Society for Artificial Internal Organs American Society for Artificial Internal Organs* 1960, 6: 104–107.

Thompson, Gilbert, ed., *Pioneers of Medicine without a Nobel Prize,* London: Imperial College Press, 2014.

Webster, Andrew, ed., *New Technologies in Health Care: Challenge, Change and Innovation,* New York: Palgrave MacMillan, 2006.

Endoscopy

What	Technology for examining a hollow organ or body cavity by means of a flexible tube equipped with optical lenses and an internal light source.
Where	Germany; France; Russia; United States
When	1806; 1853; 1901; 1957; 1980
By Whom	Philipp Bozzini (1773–1809); Antonin Desormeaux (1815–1881); Dimitri Ott (1855–1929); Basil Hirschowitz (1925–2013); Kurt Semm (1927–2003)
Importance	Major diagnostic and therapeutic innovation; makes possible minimally invasive surgical treatment of many internal diseases.

The word *endoscopy,* looking inside, is derived from the Greek *endo* (within) and *skopein* (to view). In medicine, looking inside the body goes back to ancient Greece where Hippocratic physicians employed spoonlike dilators to examine patients' natural orifices. The vaginal speculum was widely used by medieval Islamic physicians; 10th-century surgeon Albucasis reportedly used a glass mirror to reflect light for internal inspection of the cervix. For diagnosis of foreign bodies in the ear, 13th-century Guy de Chauliac recommended inspection with an aural speculum for widening the outer canal.

Modern endoscopy emerged in the early 1800s when German physician-obstetrician Philipp Bozzini developed a "light conductor" (*Lichtleiter*) to illuminate the internal parts to be examined. His device, two parallel tubes with angulated mirrors, used a candle housed in its hollow handle as a light source. The mechanical part of the instrument could be adapted to the anatomy of body orifices. In 1806 Bozzini published a description of his "invention for viewing internal parts and diseases" where he detailed its uses in physiological and pathological conditions: to inspect the urethra, rectum, and the female urinary bladder; and to assess deep abscesses, wounds, growths, and disorders of the ear, nose, mouth, vagina, and cervix. His instrument helped localize bladder stones for surgical excision and identify the source of vaginal bleeding after childbirth. Bozzini even observed the vaginal and cervical changes in female orgasm and speculated on their role in conception and female infertility. However, except for army hospital physicians, few colleagues showed interest in his device. The conservative Medical Faculty of Vienna dismissed it as another "new toy" and censored him for "undue curiosity."

Bozzini died prematurely, but until the late 1800s attempts at endoscopy were largely based on his principle. In 1853 French surgeon Antonin Desormeaux demonstrated to the Paris Medical Academy a tubular device with reconfigured mirrors and lenses and a light generated by a mixture of alcohol and turpentine that burned brighter than candlelight. Desormeaux used it to examine the urethra and bladder and coined the term "endoscopy."

In the late 1800s, German scientists further refined the technique. Maximilian Nitze, in 1879, was the first to introduce an artificial light source inside the body. His "cystoscope" had an incandescent platinum wire within a small glass sleeve that was passed via a tube and followed by a telescopic lens; the platinum wire was later replaced with the electrical wire of Edison's filament lamp. Nitze worked with opticians to construct lenses small enough to allow safe and painless introduction of his instrument. In 1881, Polish surgeon Jan Mikulicz-Radecki devised an early gastroscope to visualize the stomach by passing a rigid tube through the esophagus; the apparatus was complex and cumbersome, requiring pharyngeal anesthesia and suction to manage salivary secretions. Still, adequate illumination remained the chief practical problem in endoscopy. Burns were the most common complication.

In 1901 Dimitri Ott, founder of endoscopic surgery in Russia and physician to Tsarina Alexandra, performed the first documented abdominal examination via transvaginal access. Through an incision in the vaginal cul-de-sac he inspected the abdominal cavity using a speculum and head reflector lamp; an added light source was connected to the speculum. He called his procedure "ventroscopy." The same year Georg Kelling in Dresden experimented with high-pressure insufflation of the peritoneal cavity as a way to halt intra-abdominal bleeding, a technique he called air tamponade. He carried out numerous procedures on live dogs, introducing a Nitze cystoscope directly through a small incision in the abdominal wall to observe the effects of his method. His system, an insufflation needle and air pump with an optic trocar and telescope, laid the foundation for future diagnostic and therapeutic procedures in closed body cavities.

It was Swedish physician Hans Christian Jacobaeus who in 1910 applied the percutaneous technique to human subjects, using an artificial pneumothorax and pneumoperitoneum to evacuate ascites in tuberculous peritonitis. He called his technique "laparo-thorascopy" (from the Greek, *lapara,* flank). The following year Bertram Bernheim at Johns Hopkins University reported the first human diagnostic "organoscopy" in the United States.

Early 20th-century laparoscopy had a substantial complication rate, including intra-abdominal burns, organ puncture or rupture, and air embolism due to excessive insufflation. French gynecologist Raoul Palmer was among the first to recognize the critical importance of pressure monitoring. He also advocated the use of carbon dioxide gas (nonflammable and readily absorbed by the body) instead of atmospheric oxygen.

Other technical advances included pyramidal trocars for port placement, improved lenses, and specialized spring-loaded needles that could be blunted after introduction. In Berlin in 1936, Rudolph Schindler introduced the first semiflexible gastroscope; his device was safer and more effective and was widely adopted. German gastroenterologist Heinz Kalk in the early 1940s perfected the technique of laparoscopic liver biopsy with a wide-angle lens system. He carried out multiple procedures with no fatalities, contributing to the acceptance of laparoscopy in the diagnosis of liver disease.

The introduction of endoscopy into the field of general surgery has been relatively recent. A major technological advance was the development of a safer light source in the 1950s by Paris physician Max Fourestier. He introduced a rigid quartz light rod, which allowed transmission of abundant light while producing minimal heat. This was the breakthrough that set the stage for flexible fiber-optic technology still used in modern instruments.

In 1957, gastroenterologist Basil Hirschowitz at the University of Michigan performed the first flexible fiber-optic endoscopy when he passed his "fiberscope" down his own throat. By 1960, the American Cystoscope Manufacturing Company had produced a commercial model, offering a solution to the basic problems of optics, illumination, and tube flexibility. With an array of long, thin, tightly packed fiberglass threads that transmitted light, a magnifying lens at one end, and an eyepiece at the other, the new instrument was fully flexible and easily inserted. It greatly improved the surgeon's visual scope, and its flexibility and reduced size increased patient comfort and safety. Other technical refinements followed, including added channels for biopsy tools, suction, or irrigation and full controlled tip deflection.

Flexible fiber-optic technology transformed endoscopy, making it increasingly safe and routine. The technique quickly expanded from gastroscopy to sigmoidoscopy, colonoscopy, bronchoscopy, arthroscopy, and other areas. Gynecologists had been early pioneers in the therapeutic use of laparoscopy for lysis of pelvic adhesions, puncture of ovarian cysts, and tubal sterilization. In 1961 Raoul Palmer described the first laparoscopic retrieval of oocytes. The 1970s saw both diagnostic and therapeutic applications multiply, including colon polypectomy using wire loop snare, removal of biliary stones, and placement of gastric feeding tubes.

In 1963, Japanese firm Olympus developed a miniature camera that could be affixed to the end of the cable, thus combining photography with endoscopy. Although these initial images were often distorted by the lens or clouded by bodily fluids, internal organs and their lesions could now be photographed and documented from within. The development of a compact electronic video camera in 1985 was another major breakthrough. Live images were acquired via a light-sensitive charge-coupling device (CCD) and focused on the chip by a small lens at the tip of the instrument. These were processed into digital signals and then converted into visual images to be projected onto television screens, enlarged, recorded, and viewed in real time from a convenient distance by all members of the surgical team. The same video cable also provided for the insertion and manipulation of surgical tools for therapeutic purposes. Digital endoscopes revolutionized the practice of both diagnostic and therapeutic procedures. They have largely replaced fiber-optic devices because of significantly higher image quality. Most modern video-endoscopes use combination technology.

Therapeutic laparoscopy, already an important part of gynecological practice, now also entered the field of general surgery. The first laparoscopic appendectomy was carried out in 1980 by gynecologist Kurt Semm. In 1985 fellow German Erich Mühe and two years later Philippe Mouret in France performed the first laparoscopic cholecystectomies. These were surgical milestones leading to rapid acceptance of new endoscopic techniques. Other minimally invasive procedures soon followed, revolutionizing surgical practice.

Today, video-assisted endoscopy is widely used not only by gastroenterologists and urologists, but also by gynecologists, orthopedists, plastic and ear/nose/throat (ENT) surgeons, and many others. Procedures include excision of tumors, removal of foreign objects, opening of blocked ducts, extraction of biliary or renal stones, reconstruction of joint surfaces and ligaments, insertion of internal drains or feeding tubes, and more. The vast majority of gallbladder extractions nowadays are laparoscopic. This "keyhole" technology has many advantages. Surgery is less invasive and can usually be performed under local anesthesia, resulting in faster recovery, smaller visible scars, and lesser expense.

Newer developments include diagnostic capsule endoscopy in which a small, pill-sized capsule containing a tiny CCD-chip camera and a light-emitting diode (LED) light is swallowed by the patient, with the goal to explore areas heretofore not accessible by traditional methods.

Bibliography and Suggested Readings

Berci, George, and Forde, Kenneth A., "History of Endoscopy: What Lessons Have We Learned from the Past?," *Surgical Endoscopy* 2000, 14(1): 5–15.

Frey, Manfred, ed., *Endoscopy and Microsurgery*, Vienna: Springer, 2001.

Litynski, Grzegorz S., "Laparoscopy—The Early Attempts: Spotlighting Georg Kelling and Hans Christian Jacobaeus." *Journal of the Society of Laparoendoscopic Surgeons* 1997, 1(1): 83–85.

Modlin, Irvin, *A Brief History of Endoscopy*, Milan: Multimedia, 2000.

Shah, Jyoti, "Endoscopy through the Ages," *British Journal of Urology International* May 2002, 89(7): 645–652.

Sircus, W., "Milestones in the Evolution of Endoscopy: A Short History," *Journal of the Royal College of Physicians of Edinburgh* 2003, 33: 124–134.

Spaner, Shelley J., and Warnock, Garth L., "A Brief History of Endoscopy, Laparoscopy, and Laparoscopic Surgery," *Journal of Laparoendoscopic & Advanced Surgical Techniques*, December 1997, 7(6): 369–373.

Van Dijck, Jose, *The Transparent Body: A Cultural Analysis of Medical Imaging*, Seattle: University of Washington Press, 2005.

Heart–Lung Machine

What	Technology allowing the bypass of the heart and lungs to circulate and oxygenate blood, and maintain organ perfusion during open-heart surgery.
Where	United States
When	1953
By Whom	John Gibbon, Jr. (1903–1973)

Importance   Major technological innovation that allowed surgical correction of congenital heart defects, valvular disease, and coronary obstructions.

The development of cardiopulmonary bypass to permit open-heart surgery is one of the most important surgical advances of the last half of the 20th century. Until then, operations that required opening of the live beating heart were doomed to failure because of extensive blood loss and the inability to maintain blood circulation and tissue oxygenation during even minor interventions. It was the elaboration of a cardiopulmonary bypass (CPB) system that could bypass the heart and lungs and mechanically pump and oxygenate blood that ultimately made possible even lengthy cardiothoracic procedures.

During cardiopulmonary bypass, the "heart–lung machine" maintains organ perfusion and tissue nourishment. A cannula in the right atrium or in one of the large afferent veins withdraws venous blood from the body. The cannula is connected to tubing filled with an isotonic solution, and the syphoned-off venous blood is filtered, cooled or warmed, and oxygenated. After oxygenation the blood is returned to the systemic circulation via another cannula, usually inserted into the ascending aorta, soon after it arises from the heart. Heparin, an anticlotting agent, is administered throughout this procedure to prevent blood clotting. The blood is also cooled to lower body temperature and to slow the basal metabolic rate and overall demand for oxygen.

The idea that organ function could be maintained through extracorporeal circulation had first been suggested in the 19th century. In 1885, German physiologist Maximilian von Frey developed an early blood oxygenation system. But until the discovery of blood types and anticoagulants in the early 1900s, surgical procedures with a heart–lung bypass apparatus were not feasible, for they required a safe reversible method of anticoagulation. The 1916 discovery of heparin, which prevents clotting, paved the way for experimental advances in whole-body perfusion; protamine, the antidote that reverses the effect of heparin, first came into clinical use in the 1930s.

Aside from a mechanical pump capable of circulating blood without destroying red blood cells, the most critical component of the heart–lung machine was the artificial oxygenator that would make possible extracorporeal oxygenation of venous blood. Oxygenators replace the function of the lungs by extracting the blood's carbon dioxide and delivering oxygen during the time that heart and lungs are at rest. The earliest such devices were bubble and film oxygenators, both "direct-contact" methods because no barrier was interposed between blood and oxygen. Later membrane oxygenators introduced a gas-permeable surface between blood and oxygen, which decreased cellular trauma and made possible more prolonged use.

Cardiac surgery began in the 1940s with only a few operations that did not require cardiopulmonary bypass, such as mitral commissurotomy (opening of calcified narrowed mitral valve leaflets) or certain temporary shunt procedures. In the later decade, several open-heart interventions for closure of atrial septal defects were attempted in human patients using deep hypothermia.

The first successful open-heart surgery with total cardiopulmonary bypass was performed by John Gibbon at Thomas Jefferson University Hospital in Philadelphia in May 1953. Gibbon had had the idea of developing a heart–lung bypass machine when in 1931, during a surgical research fellowship at Massachusetts General Hospital in Boston, he witnessed a patient under his care succumb to a massive pulmonary embolus; a last-ditch Trendelenburg embolectomy was attempted but was unsuccessful. Gibbon set out to research previous work in the field, aiming to develop an apparatus that would replace the natural circulation during emergency pulmonary embolectomy. In 1934, together with his wife Mary, he started building an early heart–lung machine. The machine filmed blood over the inner surface of a rotating cylinder within an oxygen atmosphere but had limited perfusion capacity, restricting experiments to animals no larger than cats.

After World War II, with support from then IBM president Thomas Watson, Gibbon began collaborating with company engineers. By 1952 they had developed a machine using roller pumps and a film oxygenator consisting of a series of vertical stationary wire mesh screens. Blood flowed down each side of the screens, forming a film exposed to a flow of oxygen. This machine achieved a 90 percent survival rate in dogs, and after many trials in the laboratory was tried on a 15-month old child thought to have an atrial septal defect. Sadly, the patient had been misdiagnosed and did not live. Gibbon's second operation, however, was a success. He closed an atrial septal defect in an 18-year-old woman during 26 minutes of total CPB.

Two subsequent patients died due to a combination of technical problems and misdiagnosis. Following these losses, Gibbon decided to focus on improving preoperative diagnostic services and not to attempt any more heart operations himself.

Others, however, were not deterred and carried on his work. Between 1950 and 1955 several medical centers actively engaged in developing a heart–lung machine. At the University of Toronto, William Mustard developed a system that used isolated monkey lungs as an oxygenator. At the University of Minnesota, Clarence Dennis had developed a rotating disc oxygenator, and C. Walton

Lillehei began a clinical trial in which the oxygenator was one of the patient's parents, a technique called cross-circulation. In 1955, John Kirklin at the Mayo Clinic successfully used a modified Gibbon-IBM mechanical pump oxygenator to operate on eight patients, half of whom survived. Around the same time, Lillehei and his team designed their own mechanical heart–lung bypass system, the DeWall Bubble Oxygenator. Together with other research groups, these pioneer surgeons paved the way for clinical implementation of cardiopulmonary bypass in open-heart surgery.

Early operations were primarily aimed at treating congenital heart disease. In the 1960s the advent of effective artificial heart valves expanded the use of CPB to include surgical repair of acquired valvular disease. In the end, it was the introduction of coronary artery bypass grafting (CABG) in the late 1960s that led to significant increase of open-heart cardiac procedures with CPB.

Unfortunately, until the 1980s complications were numerous. Air embolism and postoperative hemorrhage were common problems. An important technological improvement was the introduction in the 1970s of cold, low-potassium cardioplegia, instead of the earlier high concentrations used to induce cardiac arrest. Suction procedures when opening the heart cavity were also identified as a major source of small emboli. This led to an effort to eliminate cardiotomy suction whenever possible, or to preprocess suctioned blood prior to returning it to the extracorporeal circulation.

The prevention of large air emboli was another serious concern. Most heart–lung machines included an arterial line bubble trap to reduce that risk. Recognition of the danger of microemboli led to the development of screen microfilters, shown to improve outcome especially when used with bubble oxygenators. Film and disc oxygenators were gradually replaced by disposable bubble oxygenators, which contained a defoaming chamber and a heat exchanger. In the mid-1980s, high-performance microporous membrane oxygenators became available; they are still the most common oxygenator in use today.

With continued technological refinements, the heart–lung machine evolved from Gibbon's highly complex, expensive apparatus, described as being the size of a grand piano, to a smaller simpler device operated by full-time specially trained perfusionists (extracorporeal technologists). Recognized as a profession in 1978, perfusionists participate in hundreds of thousands of operations using CPB every year.

Today, technological refinements, improved surgical techniques, and sophisticated cardiac diagnostic methods have come together to establish the routine use of cardiopulmonary bypass in open-heart surgery and to make it safe and effective. CPB has also fostered many other advances in critical care, including extracorporeal respiratory support, ventricular assist devices, and total artificial hearts.

Since the first operation using cardiopulmonary bypass, mortality has decreased rapidly. Death rates for many open-heart procedures now range in the single digits, with some as low as 1 percent. Cecelia Bavolek, the 18-year-old who survived Dr. Gibbon's historical surgery, remained alive and well for another 47 years; she died in the year 2000.

Bibliography and Suggested Readings

Cooper, David, *Open Heart: The Radical Surgeons Who Revolutionized Medicine*, New York: Kaplan, 2010.

Fye, Bruce, *Caring for the Heart: Mayo Clinic and the Rise of Specialization*, Oxford, New York: Oxford University Press, 2015.

Hessel, Eugene, "A Brief History of Cardiopulmonary Bypass," *Seminars in Cardiothoracic and Vascular Anesthesia* 2014, 18(2): 87–100.

Passaroni, Andréia C., et al., "Cardiopulmonary Bypass: Development of John Gibbon's Heart-Lung Machine," *Revista Brasileira de Cirurgia Cardiovascular* 2015, 30(2): 235–245.

Shumacker, Harris, *The Evolution of Cardiac Surgery*, Bloomington: Indiana University Press, 1992.

Stoney, William S., "Historical Perspectives in Cardiology: Evolution of Cardiopulmonary Bypass," *Circulation* 2009, 119: 2844–2853.

Zimmer, Heinz-Gerd, "The Heart-Lung Machine Was Invented Twice—The First Time by Max von Frey," *Clinical Cardiology* 2003, 26: 443–445.

In Vitro Fertilization (IVF)

What	Technique to assist reproduction, in which eggs removed from a woman's ovaries and fertilized by sperm "in vitro" (from the Latin, "in glass") are then implanted in the female reproductive tract.
Where	United States; United Kingdom; Australia
When	1944; 1969; 1978; 1980
By Whom	John Rock (1890–1984); Robert Edwards (1925–2013); Patrick Steptoe (1913–1988); Carl Wood (1929–2011)
Importance	Revolutionized the field of human reproduction by making possible the growth of embryos outside the body to treat infertility; established the field of reproductive medicine.

Worldwide, infertility affects more than 10 percent of all couples. In the past, the ability to help such couples was limited. The process of reproduction was mysterious, and scientific knowledge of reproductive cycles, fertilization, and embryonic development had long remained inadequate. It was not until the 19th-century discovery of the mammalian oocyte (egg cell) and the subsequent observations of early development that traditional theories of preformation—the idea that a miniature, fully preformed person was present in the male or female reproductive organ—gave way to modern embryological concepts. Research progress was also hindered by the nature and site of impregnation, egg fertilization, and embryonic development, none of which could readily be studied in their human maternal environment.

Today, on the contrary, if a woman has difficulty conceiving, reproductive endocrinologists can visualize her reproductive organs with minimally invasive laparoscopic techniques, using only tiny abdominal incisions. If she is not ovulating regularly, hormonal drugs are given to stimulate egg development. If her infertility is the result of irreversible blockage of the Fallopian tubes, in vitro fertilization is the standard of treatment. Whenever sperm and egg cannot meet inside the body, IVF has become established therapy.

Boston physician John Rock, the director of Harvard's sterility clinic, was an early pioneer in the field. His work on contraception laid the foundation for modern-day infertility treatment. In the 1930s, shortly after estrogen and progesterone had been isolated, Rock developed a procedure to analyze and "date" the lining of uterine tissue. This allowed clinicians to determine the time of ovulation, a crucial piece of information for any future reproductive technology. From 1938 until 1950, Rock conducted clinical experiments on nearly 1,000 women; he recovered 34 fertilized ova and embryos at different stages, representing the first 17 days of life. Rock and pathologist Arthur Hertig's photographs documenting these earliest phases of pregnancy constitute the first visual record of embryonic development. Their work became essential in elucidating the process of human reproduction. It captured the process of fertilization at its inception, from the descent of the ovum through the Fallopian tube to the initial cell division of the fertilized egg and its implantation in the womb.

Rock knew that if a human egg could be fertilized *in vitro* and then implanted, the widespread, often untreatable, problem of blocked oviducts could be bypassed. "What a boon for the barren woman with closed tubes!" he wrote in a 1937 *New England Journal of Medicine* editorial. In 1944, he and longtime research assistant Miriam Menkin achieved the first successful *in vitro* fertilization of human eggs. Rock and Menkin had retrieved ova from nearly 300 infertility patients undergoing diagnostic laparotomies. Menkin attempted to fertilize a total of 138 eggs, incubating them overnight and adding spermatozoa the next day; the sperm used was "leftover" semen from samples for artificial insemination. Between February and April 1944, she succeeded in fertilizing four eggs from three different women. Thus, pregnancy through *in vitro* fertilization was "not beyond the realm of imagination." Nevertheless, much additional research would be needed for a two-cell zygote to become an implantable embryo and grow into a baby.

By the late 1950s and early 1960s researchers reported the first successful IVF pregnancies in rabbits, mice, and hamsters. Much of this success hinged on the 1951 discovery by Colin R. Austin and M. C. Chang of so-called sperm capacitation, namely the changes that spermatozoa had to undergo to make them capable of fertilizing an ovum. These changes must take place, whether *in vivo* or *in vitro*, for sperm to acquire the ability to penetrate the egg's protective external membrane. The exact stimuli and molecular processes involved in capacitation are still unknown.

In the 1960s, building on the work of Rock and others, British physiologist Robert Edwards (who had been Austin's student) and gynecologist Patrick Steptoe undertook human IVF studies. Their goal was to place an egg fertilized in a Petri dish into the mother's uterus for implantation and development. Earlier, while at Johns Hopkins Hospital, Edwards had studied the initial stages of embryonic development: how human eggs mature, how different hormones regulate their maturation, at which point the eggs are receptive to the fertilizing sperm, and under which conditions sperm are activated and capacitated. He continued his work at Cambridge University and by 1969, together with Steptoe, achieved the successful *in vitro* fertilization of 13 out of 56 human eggs. Edwards devised the appropriate culture media to allow fertilization and early embryonic growth. Steptoe utilized laparoscopy to retrieve mature eggs from the ovaries of patients with tubal infertility and was instrumental in helping to move IVF from the laboratory bench to the bedside.

By 1970 Edwards and Steptoe were able to report successful embryonic development to the 16-cell stage. Seven years later, in 1977, they succeeded in establishing a pregnancy in a woman who had failed to conceive for the preceding nine years. The world's first "test-tube baby," Louise Brown, was delivered by cesarean section after a full-term pregnancy in July 1978. A second IVF birth followed soon after in 1980 with rival Australian group Alex Lopata and collaborators at Monash University, and in the United States in 1981 by IVF pioneers Howard and Georgeanna Jones at Eastern Virginia Medical School.

The birth of Louise Brown, the world's first "test-tube baby," on July 25, 1978, made medical history. Patrick Steptoe and Robert Edwards, whose work made it possible, reported clinical details in their letter to The Lancet the following month. Their groundbreaking achievement gave new hope to infertile couples around the world.

Birth after Reimplantation of a Human Embryo

"We wish to report that 1 of our patients, a 30-year-old nulliparous married woman, was safely delivered by cesarean section on July 25, 1978, of a normal healthy infant girl weighing 2700 g. The patient had been referred to one of us (P.C.S.) in 1976 with a history of 9 years' infertility, tubal occlusions, and unsuccessful salpingostomies done in 1970 with excision of the ampullae of both oviducts followed by persistent tubal blockages. Laparoscopy in February, 1977, revealed grossly distorted tubal remnants with occlusion and peritubal and ovarian adhesions. Laparotomy in August 1977, was done with excision of the remains of both tubes, adhesolysis, and suspension of the ovaries in good position for oocyte recovery. Pregnancy was established after laparoscopic recovery of an oocyte on November 10, 1977, in-vitro fertilization and normal cleavage in culture media, and the reimplantation of the 8-cell embryo into the uterus 2 1/2 days later.

Amniocentesis at 16 weeks' pregnancy revealed normal alpha-fetoprotein levels with no chromosome abnormalities in a 46 XX fetus. On the day of delivery the mother was 38 weeks and 5 days by dates from her last menstrual period, and she had preeclamptic toxemia. Blood pressure was fluctuating around 140/95, edema involved both legs up to knee level together with the abdomen, back, hands, and face. . . . Ultrasonic scanning and radiographic appearances showed that the fetus had grown slowly for several weeks from week 30. Blood-estriols and human placental lactogen levels also dropped below the normal levels during this period. However, the fetus grew considerably during the last 10 days before delivery while placental function improved greatly. On the day of delivery the biparietal diameter had reached 9.6 cm, and 5 ml of amniotic fluid was safely removed under sonic control. The lecithin:sphingomyelin ratio was . . . indicative of maturity and a low risk of the respiratory-distress syndrome. We hope to publish further medical and scientific details in your columns at a later date."

Source: Reprinted from Steptoe, P.C., and Edwards, R. G. *Lancet* August 12, 1978, 2(8085): 366, with permission from Elsevier.

In 1980, Edwards and Steptoe founded the first IVF program for infertile patients at Bourn Hall Clinic in Cambridge. Scientists from around the world came to train with them. Continuing technological refinements increased pregnancy rates. New vaginal ultrasound techniques helped identify mature eggs, which were then aspirated through a fine needle syringe instead of retrieved through laparoscopy. Innovations such as intracytoplasmic sperm injection (ICSI), where a single sperm cell is injected directly into the egg, helped improve treatment of male infertility. Other important applications included pre-implantation genetic diagnosis and gestational surrogacy, as well as derivation of human embryonic stem cells. The Australian IVF group led by Carl Wood soon became international leaders in the field, making possible a first frozen embryo pregnancy and the first surrogate birth.

Today, advances in assisted reproduction have made IVF almost routine for certain types of infertility. Women with premature ovarian failure or past their reproductive years can avail themselves of donor eggs and even donor embryos. By 2010 an estimated 4 million IVF children were alive worldwide, including nearly 200,000 born of donated eggs or embryos. In the United States approximately 58,000 IVF babies are delivered each year. IVF has proven to be safe and effective, with only rare complications; 20 percent to 30 percent of fertilized eggs lead to the birth of a child.

Initially, IVF research had met with significant hostility from various quarters, including legal actions and refusal of funding. Its advent raised ethical questions about the rights and uses of artificially produced embryos and the moral issues surrounding surrogate parenting. In the United Kingdom, the Warnock Committee in 1982 supported the use of IVF as an acceptable procedure for infertile women but advised against extra-uterine maintenance of embryos for longer than 14 days. The Catholic Church, however, opposed IVF, and some countries outlawed surrogate pregnancies. Nevertheless, in 2016 IVF is a well-established technology throughout the world, with important applications in a number of fields. IVF makes possible the production of embryos not only to treat human infertility, but also for research purposes, animal breeding, and conservation of endangered mammals.

Robert Edwards was awarded the 2010 Nobel Prize in Medicine for his pioneering work in the development of *in vitro* fertilization; Dr. Steptoe had died in 1988. The prize was the first in Nobel history to recognize the area of reproduction. Follow-up studies showing that IVF children are as healthy as normally conceived children were a contributing factor for conferring the long-delayed award.

Bibliography and Suggested Readings

Bavister, Barry D., "Early History of In Vitro Fertilization," *Reproduction* 2002, 124: 181–196.

Clarke, Gary, "A.R.T. and History," *Human Reproduction* 2006, 21(7): 1645–1650.

Deech, Ruth, and Smajdor, Anna, *From IVF to Immortality: Controversy in the Era of Reproductive Technology*, Oxford: Oxford University Press: 2007.

Leeton, John, *Test Tube Revolution: The Early History of IVF*, Clayton: Monash University Publishing, 2013.

Marsh, Margaret, and Ronner, Wanda, *The Fertility Doctor: John Rock and the Reproductive Revolution*, Baltimore: Johns Hopkins University Press, 2008.

Pfeffer, Naomi, "Pioneers of Infertility Treatment," in *Women and Modern Medicine*, eds. Lawrence Conrad and Anne Hardy, Amsterdam: Brill, Rodopi, 2001, pp. 245–261.

Rock, John, and Menkin, Miriam F., "In Vitro Fertilization and Cleavage of Human Ovarian Eggs," *Science* August 4, 1944, 100(2588): 105–107.

Steptoe, Patrick C., and Edwards, Robert G., "Birth after the Reimplantation of a Human Embryo," *Lancet* 1978, 2(8085): 366.

Organ Transplantation

What	The implanting of a healthy vital organ or tissue from one body to another in order to replace a diseased or failing one.
Where	United Kingdom; United States; France
When	1902; 1905; 1954; later
By Whom	Alexis Carrel (1873–1944); Peter Medawar (1915–1987); Frank Macfarlane Burnet (1899–1985); Joseph E. Murray (1919–2012); E. Donnall Thomas (1920–2012); Jean Dausset (1916–2009); many others
Importance	Major surgical innovation of the 20th century that prolonged thousands of lives; often the only treatment for patients with end-stage organ failure.

Surgical interest in reconstructing diseased or defective body parts has a long history, as do cultural myths of successful magical replacement of lost tissues and limbs. Ancient medical manuscripts from the sixth century B.C. describe procedures grafting skin flaps to repair nose amputations. The twin surgeons and early Christian martyrs, Cosmas and Damian, were credited with the miraculous replacement of an ulcerated limb, and generated an abundant iconography. Sixteenth-century surgeon Gaspare Tagliacozzi built his reputation on careful rhinoplasties, in which he transferred to the patient's nasal stump healthy tissue from another part of the body; an illustrated 1597 treatise *"On the surgery of mutilation by grafting"* detailed his methods. In England, John Hunter (1728–1793) conducted numerous transplant experiments with animals. He also studied human tooth transplantation, traditionally performed by barber-surgeons. Public fascination with these early attempts at plastic and transplant surgery contributed to inspiring a new genre of science fiction, including Mary Shelley's 1831 novel *Frankenstein*.

A key figure in the early history of transplant medicine was French surgeon Alexis Carrel. In 1902, he perfected a reliable method for connecting arteries

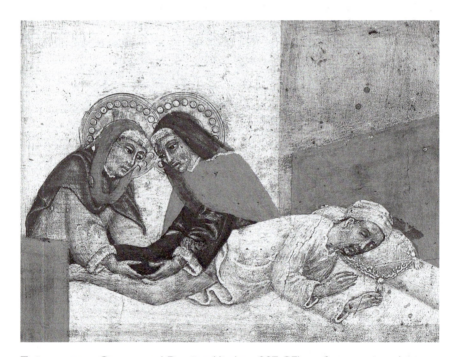

Twin surgeons Cosmas and Damian (died ca. 287 CE) perform a miraculous cure by grafting a recently deceased man's leg to replace a gangrenous limb (painting by Sano di Pietro, 1405–1481). According to legend, the brothers were highly skilled doctors who practiced without charging a fee for their services. They are regarded as patron saints of physicians in Catholic and Orthodox Christian belief. (DeAgostini/Getty Images)

and veins by end-to-end vascular anastomosis; this not only protected against postoperative bleeding or clotting, but also prevented constriction of the suture site. Carrel reportedly learned his delicate stitching techniques from professional silk embroiderers in his native Lyon. His work, which also included cold storage tissue preservation, was recognized with the 1912 Nobel Prize in Physiology or Medicine. He had made organ grafting technically feasible.

Still, successful transplantation remained beyond reach for transplants were almost inevitably rejected. The recipient's body fought the new organ just as it would a disease. It was not until the 1950s that some of the underlying immunological mechanisms were understood.

In the early years of transplant medicine, corneal grafting had been the only procedure to succeed. Because the cornea has no blood supply, circulating lymphocytes did not reach the graft to reject it; Viennese ophthalmologist Eduard Zirm in 1905 had carried out a first successful full-thickness corneal transplant, restoring sight to a 45-year-old laborer accidentally blinded by caustic lime.

In the 1940s British biologist Peter Medawar developed the concept of "active acquired immunity" that explained the repeated loss of skin grafts in burn victims. In 1953 he discovered the existence of another powerful mechanism—that of immunologic tolerance; this, too, could be acquired and potentially used to advantage in organ and tissue transplants. Medawar demonstrated his theory in a famous study in which donor cells from adult mice were injected into fetuses of a different genetic strain; once adult, the injected mice had become "tolerant" to skin grafts from the original donors. Medawar's work extended the findings of Australian scientist Macfarlane Burnet that the fetus would recognize as "self" all foreign tissue encountered prenatally and therefore not mount an antibody response. Medawar and Burnet earned the 1960 Nobel Prize for their work on the "*discovery of acquired immunological tolerance.*"

The first organ to be successfully transplanted was the kidney. Kidneys were relatively easy to remove and moreover could be harvested from living donors because only one kidney is needed to preserve full renal function. Experimental allografts had been performed in dogs since the early 1900s. Human-to-human transplants had been attempted first by pioneer Soviet surgeon Voronoy in 1933, then by a number of French and U.S. surgeons. However, all failed because of transplant rejection. In 1954, Boston surgeons Joseph Murray and David Hume carried out the first successful kidney transplant between 23-year-old homozygous twins shown to be identical by fingerprinting and skin grafting, thus being immunologically compatible. The recipient, Richard Herrick, who was dying of acute glomerulonephritis, married his nurse and lived another eight years.

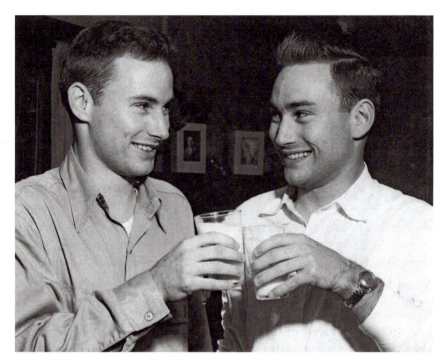

Identical twins Ronald (left) and Richard Herrick celebrate a few months after Ronald donated one of his kidneys to Richard in the world's first successful kidney transplant in 1954. Richard lived for another eight years after the operation. His brother Ronald died in 2010 of complications following heart surgery. (Jack Sheahan/The Boston Globe/Getty Images)

The success of the Herrick operation ushered in a new era. In 1959 two successful kidney transplants were performed between nontwinned siblings, using low-dose radiation preoperatively to suppress recipient immunity. In 1962, Jean Hamburger's Paris team performed the first successful transplant of an extended family donor selected using early tissue-typing methods. Pretreatment with radiation was abandoned in favor of chemical immunosuppression. Nevertheless, overall results were poor.

By the 1970s important insights into the physiological and pathological functions of the kidney had been gained. At the same time, researchers had gradually elucidated the "biological force" in organ rejection as an immunological defense mechanism mediated by lymphocytes. During the 1950s and 1960s, scientists Benacerraf, Dausset, and Snell—later to become joint Nobel laureates—discovered the existence of specific, genetically determined substances on the white cell surface, which regulate immunological reactions. They were termed human leukocyte antigens (HLAs).

In transplants, HLA antigens are recognized by the recipient's immune system as foreign and thus rejected. When immunologically active donor cells are transplanted, they in turn recognize the recipient's cells as foreign and destroy them. This was what led to the frequently fatal "graft vs. host" (GVH) reactions. Controlling these reactions during transplantation was essential to avoid graft rejection or GVH disease. Corticosteroids, radiation, and antimetabolites or cytotoxic drugs such as azathioprine and methotrexate (also used as cancer drugs), all suppressed the immune response, thus diminishing the risk of rejection. Until the discovery of cyclosporine in the late 1970s, maintenance immunosuppression with a combination of azathioprine and high-dose cortisone proved best in treating graft rejection.

Joseph Murray, Richard Herrick's surgeon, who during World War II had been faced with the challenges of skin graft loss at Valley Forge Army Hospital's burn unit, became an international leader in the study of mechanisms of rejection and the use of immunosuppressive agents. He was awarded a Nobel Prize in 1990 for his work. The award also recognized E. Donnall Thomas who in 1968 had performed the first successful bone marrow transplant using the cytotoxic drug methotrexate.

The success of renal transplants in the 1950s paved the way for other human organ transplants. In 1963 James Hardy in Mississippi performed the first successful lung transplant; the same year Thomas Starzl of the University of Colorado successfully transplanted a human liver. In 1967, South African surgeon Christiaan Barnard implanted the heart of a 23-year-old accident victim into 54-year-old Louis Washkansky at Groote Schuur Hospital in Cape Town; the immunosuppressed patient succumbed to pneumonia 18 days later. The following year, Norman Shumway and Denton Cooley performed successive heart transplants in the United States; survival was 15 days and seven months, respectively. Nearly 200 heart transplants were performed during the next few years; however, most patients died shortly after transplant.

By the 1980s, the discovery of cyclosporine together with tissue typing and HLA donor-recipient crossmatching became major breakthroughs in the field, establishing the lasting success of transplant medicine. Tissue typing, developed at UCLA in 1964 by Paul Terasaki to evaluate donor and recipient HLA compatibility, became the international standard for transplant matching. Cyclosporine, a compound produced by soil fungi and discovered in 1978, selectively suppressed T-cells; given in conjunction with steroids, it prevented transplant rejection. Tacrolimus (Prograf), an even more potent soil fungus derivative, was developed a few years later and approved for clinical use in 1994.

By then, transplants included lung, liver, small bowel, and pancreatic islet cells. In 1998 a first successful hand transplant was performed in France, followed in 2005 by a partial face transplant. The introduction of laparoscopic surgery in the 1990s made organ donation by living donors simpler and easier, reducing pain and hospital stays. One- and five-year survival rates for transplanted organs continued to rise thanks to specific HLA matching and better immunosuppressive drugs. In the United States, there are now each year over 20,000 organ transplants and nearly 800,000 tissue transplants. Worldwide, transplant patients are numbered in the millions.

Although the history of transplantation is one of extraordinary progress where better understanding of human physiology and immunology opened up new ways to combat disease, transplantation medicine has remained among the most challenging areas of modern medicine. Chronic immunosuppression to prevent organ rejection has many harmful side effects, including the risk of life-threatening opportunistic infections. Nonetheless, and in spite of high economic costs, public opinion and policy generally support organ donation; the main constraint to transplantation remains procurement of donor tissues and shortage of live or cadaveric donors. As of December 2014, the waiting list for organ transplants compiled by the U.S. Department of Health and Human Services included over 120,000 patients.

Bibliography and Suggested Readings

Hamilton, David, *A History of Organ Transplantation: Ancient Legends to Modern Practice*, Pittsburgh: University of Pittsburgh Press, 2012.

Organ Procurement and Transplantation Network, http://optn.transplant.hrsa.gov.

Tilney, Nicholas L., *Transplant: From Myth to Reality*, New Haven: Yale University Press, 2003.

Pacemaker

What	Electronic device delivering rhythmic electrical impulses to the heart to restore myocardial contraction, regulate heart rate, and reestablish cardiac function in the case of arrest or life-threatening arrhythmia.
Where	United States; Canada; Sweden
When	1932; 1952; 1958
By Whom	Albert Hyman (1893–1972); Paul Zoll (1911–1999); Earl Bakken (1924–); Rune Elmqvist (1906–1997); Åke Senning (1915–2000)

Importance   Major technological innovation treating abnormalities of the electrical conduction system of the heart muscle.

The development of artificial pacemakers transformed the treatment of heart disease. As understanding of cardiac physiology advanced, it became clear that failure of the electrical conduction system of the heart, the heart's natural pacemaker, led to slowing or irregularity of the heartbeat or even cardiac arrest. Such conduction problems were common in elderly patients and a frequent complication of heart attacks, when scarred muscle tissue interferes with the transmission of the electrical impulse. Different therapeutic challenges emerged: the need for defibrillation, restoring the synchronous pumping of a quivering heart, restarting a stopped heartbeat, and correcting a rate that was either too fast or too slow to maintain adequate cardiac output.

The idea of an outside source of electricity to stimulate the heart was based on the discovery that myocardial tissue generates electrical impulses. Scottish surgeon John Hunter in the late 18th century was the first to recommend electrical resuscitation of drowning victims. In the late 19th century scientists discovered that electric shock could restart a stopped heart. Physiologist John MacWilliam in 1899 proposed that ventricular fibrillation—the most common cause of sudden death—could be terminated by a series of pulsed electrical stimuli. He suggested external pacing to treat cardiac arrest and demonstrated that applying rhythmic impulses would regulate the heart rate. This work laid the foundations for the future field of electrophysiology and the development of the artificial cardiac pacemaker.

American cardiologist Albert Hyman in the early 1930s was first to investigate electrical methods for restarting the heart after arrest. He had tried intracardiac injection of various medications but quickly realized that it was the injecting needle as it punctured the cardiac wall that set off the current that restarted contractions. From 1930 to 1932, with his engineer brother, he developed an electromechanical device designed specifically for cardiac resuscitation. The apparatus transmitted an electrical impulse to the heart by means of a needle electrode inserted through the chest wall into the patient's right atrium. Heavy and bulky, it was powered by a spring-wound motor, which turned a magnet to generate current and was operated by a hand crank. Pacing could be delivered at rates of 30, 60, or 120 impulses per minute for about six minutes. But Hyman's "artificial pacemaker" was plagued by technical difficulties. It was also considered too invasive and faced considerable opposition by the medical community, which dismissed it as dangerous "gadgetry" trying to interfere with nature.

In the late 1940s Toronto cardiothoracic surgeons Wilfred Bigelow and John Callaghan began experimenting with stimulation of the sinoatrial node (the heart's natural pacemaker) to treat cardiac arrest, a frequent result of hypothermia induced during heart surgery. With the help of engineer John Hopps they designed an endocardial electrode that was threaded into the right atrium through the external jugular vein and powered by an external vacuum-tube device.

Their work inspired Boston cardiologist Paul Zoll, who had been experimenting with defibrillation techniques, to develop a pacemaking apparatus. Having only limited technical knowledge, Zoll used a commercially available electrical pulse stimulator. Instead of an esophageal electrode, difficult to insert in emergencies, he resorted to just two external chest electrodes held in place by a leather strap on either side of the heart. However, because the electrodes were not in direct contact with the heart muscle, a strong voltage stimulus was required to capture the heartbeat and drive the ventricles. This could be painful or cause local burns.

Zoll's approach was novel but effective, "it just took a large current." He first made successful use of his closed-chest bedside treatment in a 65-year-old man with Stokes-Adams syndrome, a condition leading to recurrent cardiac arrest. In November 1952, the *New England Journal of Medicine* published the report of his "quick, simple, effective and safe method of arousing the heart from ventricular standstill by an artificial, external, electric pacemaker." Zoll kept his patient alive during ventricular asystole for several days. After discharge, the man survived for another 10 months.

Zoll's pacemaker had serious practical drawbacks but brought together existing medical and technological knowledge to solve a clinical problem: it was effective in stimulating the ventricles to contract. Pacing the ventricle rather than the atrium had been an important insight. The external pacemaker gained relatively rapid acceptance. It was easy, noninvasive, and produced quick, dramatic results. It was Zoll's innovation that led to the recognition of artificial pacemaking as a viable method of emergency resuscitation and stimulated future research.

By late 1950s hospitals were increasingly adding advanced therapeutic technologies to the routine use of X-ray and electrocardiogram (ECG). Cardiac pacing became one of them, and was to be closely associated with open-heart surgery. At the University of Minnesota surgeons started experimenting with acute cardiac pacing to treat postoperative heart block, a common and invariably fatal complication occurring when the heart's conductive tissue was damaged during surgery. C. Walton Lillehei, a pioneer in repair of ventricular septal defects, believed that with enough time the conduction system of a child with heart block would heal naturally. External pacing was impracticable because his small patients could not tolerate the intense repetitive shocks. In the end Lillehei and his team came up with the idea of implanting an electrode that would actually touch the surface of the heart. By delivering electrical stimulation directly to the excitable tissue, they might capture the heartbeat at a much lower voltage.

Their myocardial pacing wire was the first implanted electrical device. Made of silver-plated braided copper encased in a Teflon sleeve, it was inserted in the wall of the left ventricle, tied down, and brought out through the surgical incision. A second electrode was buried under the skin, and both were connected to an external pulse generator. In this way children could be paced for days or weeks after heart surgery. Lillehei found that when the heart's natural pacemaker resumed control, he could pull gently on the wire and draw it out without reopening the chest. By late 1957, the technique had been used successfully in 18 patients.

Still, this modified Zoll system remained cumbersome for it had to be plugged into an outlet, keeping the children tethered to the hospital electrical system. Possible power surges or power failures were additional concerns. Lillehei therefore asked Earl Bakken, a young engineer who serviced equipment for his department, to develop a battery-operated pacemaker. Bakken, founder of a small medical instrumentation firm called Medtronic, had been fascinated with electrical devices since childhood; as a young boy, the 1931 movie *Frankenstein* impressed him with the notion of restoring life through electricity. Using two transistors and a small nine-volt battery he built a portable pulse generator, with leads running up to the chest, an on-off switch, and controls for amplitude and rate. His first model had recessed knobs to prevent the children from changing their own heart rates, and a red neon light that blinked with each pulse; it could be strapped to the patient's chest. The new product was thus not only portable but also wearable, and Lillehei used it successfully to treat children with post-operative heart block. The Medtronic pacemaker conclusively demonstrated the safety and effectiveness of the new technology and established the company as industry leader in pacemaker manufacturing.

The next challenge was to build a fully implantable pacing device. This would allow for greater patient freedom and reduce the dangers of infection posed by running a wire from the patient's body. Such a device needed to be not only very light but also have a long-lasting energy source. In addition, its internal leads would have to conduct electrical current without harming bodily tissues.

Swedish physician-engineer Rune Elmqvist and surgeon Åke Senning in 1958 rose to this challenge, developing a device that incorporated new silicon transistors into a pulse generator small enough to harbor under the skin. They implanted two electrodes into the myocardium through a chest wall incision and channeled these to a pacemaker box in the abdominal wall. Their first pacemaker was battery powered and charged externally by an induction coil; it failed after only three hours. Their second device functioned effectively for a week. Their patient, a 43-year-old man with severe recurrent heart block, eventually underwent a total of 26 operations and received 22 pacemakers; he lived another 43 years to the age of 86.

Implantable pacemakers were further developed in the 1960s. Venous leads replaced epicardial leads, allowing pacemaker insertion without opening the chest or using general anesthesia. In 1972 American Wilson Greatbatch led the change to lithium-iodine batteries, which had a much longer life (up to 10 years), could be sealed hermetically, and were smaller and lighter.

In the mid-1970s pacemakers became programmable to patients' clinical needs through radio frequency telemetry. By the end of the decade, dual-chamber pacemakers could pace and sense both atria and ventricles. So-called "demand" pacemakers followed, which could sense underlying cardiac impulses and provide pacing only as needed.

By 1974 cardiac pacing was so widespread that the U.S. Food and Drug Administration commissioned a study on its safety and effectiveness. Their final report, issued 20 years later, emphasized pacemaker successes and improvements made since the inception of the study, many related to advances in engineering, materials, and electronics.

In the 1990s microprocessor-driven pacemakers appeared, capable of detecting cardiac events and modifying internal pacing parameters according to patient needs and activity levels. Pacing was either single or dual chamber, with electrodes implanted either in the left ventricle alone or in both right and left ventricles. Biventricular pacing for heart failure was introduced in the next decade; two electrodes were placed on opposite sides of the same ventricle to synchronize contraction and improve pump efficiency. Nowadays, sophisticated sensors detect not just heart rate and blood pressure, but also oxygen and carbon dioxide concentrations and record electrocardiograms analyzed in real time to adjust heart rate as needed.

Modern pacemakers have become light, small, long-lasting, battery-powered computers that can remedy dangerous heart conditions to improve and extend human lives. Temporary, they are used for pacing during surgery and acute care; implanted and permanent, they control cardiac rhythms in both bradycardia (slow heartbeat) and tachycardia (rapid heartbeat) syndromes. When no beat is detected, pacemakers stimulate the ventricle with a low voltage pulse;

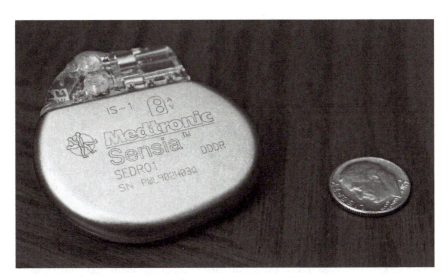

The early pacemakers, which were heavy and cumbersome, have today been replaced by light, fully-implantable miniature devices, such as this Medtronic Sensia pacemaker shown here at company headquarters in Minnesota on March 9, 2010. (Craig Lassig/Bloomberg via Getty Images)

complex units can sense activity in both atrial and ventricular chambers. Life-threatening fibrillation is treated with implantable cardioverter defibrillators (ICDs).

Hundreds of thousands of patients have benefited from pacemaker technology. By the end of the 20th century, an estimated 200,000 artificial pacemakers were implanted worldwide each year.

Bibliography and Suggested Readings

Aquilina Oscar, "A Brief History of Cardiac Pacing," *Images in Pediatric Cardiology* 2006, 8(2): 17–81.

Geselowitz, M. N., and Leder, R. S., "STARS: Pacemakers [Scanning Our Past]," *Proceedings of the IEEE* August 2013, 101(8): 1882–1888.

Jeffrey, Kirk. *Machines in Our Hearts: The Cardiac Pacemaker, the Implantable Defibrillator, and American Health Care.* Baltimore: The Johns Hopkins University Press, 2001.

Ward, Catherine, et al., "A Short History on Pacemakers," *International Journal of Cardiology* 2013, 169: 244–248.

Prosthetic Hip

What	Artificial hip joint inserted surgically to replace diseased or damaged bone or cartilage.
Where	United Kingdom; United States; France
When	1930s to 1960s
By Whom	John Charnley (1911–1982); many others
Importance	Highly successful, important advance in modern technological surgery; reduced pain from damaged hip joints, restored locomotor function, and improved quality of life; paved the way for surgical replacement of other joints.

Total hip replacement, or total hip arthroplasty, revolutionized the treatment of hip arthritis. Considered one of the most successful orthopedic procedures to date, the operation provides an effective solution for advanced osteoarthritis and other disorders of the hip joint. Such conditions are especially widespread in the elderly population, where degenerative disease leads to breakdown of bony or connective tissue. Joint surfaces become rough and uneven, causing stiffness, swelling, and pain whenever the head of the femur rubs against the hip socket. Brittle bones and fractures in the aged, as well as other inflammatory or traumatic hip disorders, can similarly lead to severe disability.

In total hip replacement (THR) the diseased cartilage and bone of the joint is replaced with artificial materials. The normal hip is a highly mobile ball-and-socket joint where the ball—the femoral head—moves within a cup-shaped socket—the acetabulum of the hip. THR entails replacement of the diseased ball and socket with a metal or ceramic ball and stem inserted into the femur (the femoral prosthesis) and an artificial metal, acrylic, or ceramic cup socket (the acetabular prosthesis). The femoral prosthesis is generally fixed into the central marrow of the femur with acrylic cement. Alternative cementless prostheses have microscopic pores to allow bone growth into the implant stem. This type of implant lasts longer and is generally used in younger patients.

Artificial hips were first developed using a variety of materials and techniques. Early operations consisted of inserting materials between articulating surfaces or of replacing one side of the hip joint. The very first procedures date back to the late 19th century when surgeons tried interposing various tissues between the articular surfaces of the arthritic hip, a technique known as interpositional arthroplasty. In 1885 Leopold Ollier in Lyon experimented with inserting adipose tissue into the joint to reduce friction and pain. Others tried muscle, celluloid, rubber, magnesium, zinc, glass, and wax. Later interpositional materials would include tendinous fascia, pig bladder, and even gold foil. Generally, however, these procedures were not effective.

In 1891 German professor Themistocles Glück developed a fixed hip implant fashioned of ivory and attached to bone with nickel-plated screws to treat patients with tubercular hip joints. Later surgeons practiced varying degrees of excisional reconstructions or advocated the less invasive removal of bony spurs from the diseased hip, a procedure known as cheilotomy. Such interventions had only limited success, for any remission of pain was at the expense of joint mobility or stability.

In 1925 Boston surgeon Marius Smith-Petersen created the first artificial interpositional arthroplasty using a hollow glass hemisphere molded over the femoral head, aiming to facilitate joint movement over a smooth biocompatible interface. Unfortunately, these glass molds failed to withstand joint pressures and often broke. Smith-Petersen went on to experiment with various other materials such as celluloid, Bakelite, and Pyrex, until 1937 when his dentist suggested he try a new alloy named Vitallium. Recently introduced to the dentistry market, Vitallium was made of cobalt, chromium, and molybdenum and was resistant to corrosion. In the following decade Smith-Petersen implanted several hundred Vitallium molds with good clinical results.

In 1938, London orthopedist Philip Wiles devised a total hip arthroplasty with fitted stainless steel implants fixed to the bone by screws and bolts, but results were unsatisfactory, because screws could loosen and unfasten the metal ball attached to the femur. Ten years later, Paris surgeons Robert and Jean Judet designed an entirely acrylic prosthesis, which was at first widely acclaimed but ultimately proved too susceptible to wear and tear. The Judets, as well as Frederick Thompson and Austin Moore in the United States, also developed metal replacements for the head of the femur. By the early 1950s, George Kenneth McKee of Norwich, England, a student of Wiles, was using wholly metallic implants on a regular basis. His prostheses had an excellent survival rate, but came into disfavor in the mid-1970s because some devices were found to cause intra-articular damage with loose metallic particles.

It was Manchester Royal Infirmary orthopedist John Charnley who pioneered the first definitive hip replacement procedure in the early 1960s. Charnley, considered the father of modern hip arthroplasty, was inspired by his experiences as an orthopedic surgeon in World War II. At that time, treatments available for fractured or severely arthritic hips were fixation (arthrodesis), which reduced pain but limited mobility; or, on the other hand, mold arthroplasties such as Smith-Petersen's and the Judets' procedures, which presented the risk of infection and/or loosening. Charnley—like many surgeons also an amateur engineer—thought that joint friction could be reduced with a femoral head implant much smaller than the bone it was replacing. Drawing on the expertise of the mechanical engineering department at Manchester's technical university, he developed a prosthesis that consisted of a stainless steel femoral stem and a polyethylene acetabular cup. To this end he employed a local fitter and turner, technician Harry Craven, who hand-made many of the parts in a workshop at Charnley's home. Prostheses were sterilized in formaldehyde overnight for use the next day and were cemented in place with pink acrylic dental cement obtained from the University of Manchester dental school.

Charnley's key innovation was use of the small femoral head, which decreased erosive wear due to its lesser surface area. He also recognized that body fluids would not adequately lubricate the implant, which led him to study a variety of lubricants, new industrial plastics, and adhesives. Clinical tests in the late 1960s demonstrated the remarkable mechanical success of his eventual design. Known as the *low friction arthroplasty*,' Charnley's metal and plastic device, with both parts cemented in, was hailed as a breakthrough in joint replacement and was taken up across the Western world. The Charnley hip was not patented and remains in extensive use today.

In the United Kingdom, the success of the Charnley prosthesis displaced nearly all other types; metal-polyethylene implants are still the most widely used and provide reliable and cost-effective outcomes for the majority of patients. In continental Europe, many hip arthroplasties use the ceramic implants introduced in 1970 by French surgeon Pierre Boutin. Tough, inert, scratch resistant, and hydrophilic, ceramic bearings increase lubrication, decrease friction, and have excellent longevity. They are preferred in young, active patients but they are much more costly. Metal-on-metal prostheses are also experiencing renewed acceptance, for prosthetic wear has proved much less than that of metal-on-polyethylene implants. The larger metal femoral heads increase joint stability, and thus incidence of dislocation; metallic implants also reduce bone breakdown and inflammatory reactions. Previous concerns about prosthetic loosening or potential carcinogenicity have been allayed; these are now attributed to poor early designs and implantation techniques.

The total hip replacement operation was a landmark advance in 20th-century surgery and played an important role in restoring mobility and alleviating pain for thousands of patients. Its development evolved from an early "cottage industry" of surgeon-inventors and engineers into a major, successful, multinational medical technology industry with a profusion of prosthetic models, which undergo constant innovative change as operators and manufacturers looked for better performance, wider application, and greater profitability. Early failures stimulated the search for improved materials and fixation methods. Antibiotics were added to bone cement to reduce infection; techniques were refined and standardized. Eventually, advances in materials and technology not only resulted in consistently reproducible and successful hip replacements, but also found new applications in the development of prostheses for other diseased joints, primarily the knee.

Today, THR has become one the most common elective surgical procedures worldwide, with thousands performed every year. In the United States in 2010, total hip replacement procedures numbered 332,000; in the United Kingdom, 2013 statistics show a total of nearly 90,000. In Europe, national registers record the success of different types of implants, measuring their survival and rates of revision.

Bibliography and Suggested Readings

Centers for Disease Control and Prevention, 2016, "Inpatient Surgery," http://www.cdc.gov/nchs/fastats/inpatient-surgery.htm.

Faulkner, Alex, "Casing the Joint: The Material Development of Artificial Hips," in *Artificial Parts, Practical Lives: Modern Histories of Prosthetics*, eds. Ott, K., Serlin, D., and Mihm, S., New York: New York University Press, 2002.

Gomez, Pablo, and Morcuende, José, "Early Attempts at Hip Arthroplasty 1700s to 1950s," *Iowa Orthopedic Journal* 2005, 25: 25–29.

Knight, Stephen Richard, Aujla, Randeep, and Biswas, Satya Prasad, "Total Hip Arthroplasty—Over 100 Years of Operative History," *Orthopedic Reviews* 2011, 3(2): e16.

Metcalfe, J. Stanley, and Pickstone, John, "Replacing Hips and Lenses: Surgery, Industry and Innovation in Post-War Britain," in *New Technologies in Health Care,* ed. Andrew Webster, London: Palgrave, 2006, pp. 146–160.

Reynolds, Lois A., and Tansey, Elizabeth M., eds., *Early Development of Total Hip Replacement, Wellcome Witnesses to Twentieth Century Medicine,* Vol. 29, London: Wellcome Trust Centre for the History of Medicine at UCL, 2007, http://www.njrreports.org.uk/hips-all-procedures-activity/H02v2NJR.

Stem Cell Therapy

What	The use of stem cells to treat disease.
Where	Canada; United Kingdom; United States; Japan
When	1960s; 1981; 1998; 2007

By Whom   Ernest McCulloch (1926–2011); James Till (1931–); Leroy Ste-
               vens (1920–2015); Martin Evans (1941–); Gail Martin (1944–);
               James Thomson (1958–); John Gurdon (1933–); Shinya
               Yamanaka (1962–)
Importance   Stem cells have enormous potential for treating disease through
               regenerative or tissue engineering techniques. Bone marrow
               transplantation, the first stem cell therapy, has cured many thou-
               sands of patients.

Long before modern stem cell therapy and bioengineering, scientists envisioned
tissue regeneration and hypothesized the existence of some type of precursor cell
in the body. The term "stem cell" first appeared in the scientific literature in 1868
when it was used by German biologist Ernst Häckel to describe both the fertilized egg that gives rise to an adult organism and the single ancestor cell of all
multicellular organisms. In the early 1900s, the concept of stem cells accounted
for the ability of blood, skin, bone, and connective tissue to self-replicate, even
though efforts to isolate these cells until then had failed. It was not until decades
later that advances in biomedical sciences led to the identification first of animal and then human stem cells. Today, stem cell therapy, together with tissue
engineering and regenerative medicine, seek to harness this knowledge to repair
or replace biological function lost because of disease, injury, or aging.

Stem cells are the cellular matrix from which all body parts are made. They
can divide to produce new copies of themselves, and new cells have the potential
to differentiate into other more specialized cell types. The human body is made
up of over 200 different types of cells, all derived from a single fertilized egg.
During embryonic development, as different tissues are formed, most cells gradually lose their stem cell properties and their ability to differentiate. The process starts when the fertilized egg transforms first into the blastocyst and then
into both specialized and stem cells for specific tissues or organs. The latter,
known as *progenitor* cells, differentiate only into cell types needed for the proper
function of their own specific organ. They exist in small numbers and, until they
are activated by disease or injury, may remain dormant for years.

Stem cells are divided into two major categories, embryonic and adult.
Embryonic stem cells are those of the early-stage embryo (the three- to five-day-
old blastocyst). Adult stem cells are found in mature tissues after birth, not only
in bone marrow, blood, brain, skin, muscle, and liver, but also in the umbilical
cord.

If a stem cell can form all cell types of both embryo and adult, including germ
cells (eggs and sperm) and placenta, it is considered *totipotent*. Examples are

the fertilized egg and some of the early blastomeres resulting from its cleavage; however, these cells do not self-renew. A stem cell that can form all cell types except extra-embryonic structures is called *pluripotent*. Embryonic stem cells are pluripotent. All other stem cells found in fetal or adult tissues are *multipotent* if they can form a variety of cell types; they are *unipotent* if they are able to form only one other cell type.

The earliest clinical use of stem cells was their extraction and transplantation from bone marrow. In 1949, after World War II and the bombing of Hiroshima, to develop treatments for radiation sickness in case of nuclear attack, American radiation expert Leon Jacobson and his colleague Egon Lorenz demonstrated how mice could be protected from the lethal effects of radiation. They encased their spleens or femurs with lead, which allowed the animals to rebuild their depleted blood supply. The researchers concluded that an active principle in the spleen or the bone marrow stimulated recovery. British biophysicist D.W.H. Barnes and others later showed this principle to be cell based.

Building on this work, Canadian scientists Ernest McCulloch and James Till at the Ontario Cancer Institute carried out a series of experiments in which they transplanted bone marrow in mice. They showed that the transplanted marrow cells induced the growth of specialized "colony-forming units" of blood cells, all derived from a single cell. These colony-forming cells in effect represented "a new class of progenitor cells." McCulloch and Till's 1961 landmark paper, followed in 1963 by co-worker Andrew Becker's, proved the existence of blood-forming stem cells and defined their fundamental properties: the capacity to differentiate into clones of specialized cells and the ability to self-replicate and perpetuate the process of differentiation. Bone marrow transplantation for leukemia, carried out since the 1950s, now had a scientific underpinning. It remains to this day the most successful clinical application of stem cell science.

The blood-forming, or *hematopoietic*, stem cells of the bone marrow were found to be the originators of all specialized blood cell types: white and red blood cells and platelets. Thus, bone marrow stem cells could be used to treat a number of hematological malignancies such as leukemia and lymphoma, where they replaced malignant bone marrow cells destroyed by chemotherapy or radiation. They served a rescue function after certain breast cancer chemotherapies, where they regenerated bone marrow depressed or depleted by cytotoxic agents.

Bone marrow was also found to contain certain osteogenic precursor cells. In 1963, A. J. Friedenstein demonstrated their existence by implanting bone marrow under the renal capsule and growing bony tissue. These cells became known as mesenchymal stem cells. Described in 1991, they could be cultured to give rise to a variety of mesenchymal tissues, including bone, cartilage, muscle, tendon, and skin. Biologist Arnold Caplan showed that bone and cartilage growth in the embryo, as well as repair and turnover in the adult, involved a small number of mesenchymal stem cells and their progeny.

This work, like that of Till and McCulloch, focused on adult stem cells. The discovery of embryonic stem cells took a separate path starting with U.S. developmental biologist Leroy Stevens's pioneering studies of germ cell tumors (teratomas) in mouse testes. His observations led him to propose that such tumors—made up of many different tissues including skin, bone, and hair—arose from abnormally proliferating pluripotent cells, which then differentiated into a variety of cell types. Stevens's pluripotent embryonic stem cells eventually became known as EC—embryonal carcinoma—cells. They could transform into normal or cancerous cells and could give rise to entire organisms.

British biochemist Martin Evans and American Gail Martin in 1981 were the first to establish that the inner cells of early normal mouse embryos could support development. They cultured mouse "embryonic stem (ES) cells" (a term coined by Martin) and developed stable cell lines capable of generating every adult tissue. Evans went on to alter the genome of mouse ES cells, developing the so-called "knock-out" technology in which homologous recombination (the exchange of DNA sequences within chromosome pairs) is used to modify specific genes. Such gene targeting, used to inactivate or modify single genes and repair or introduce mutations, has become a powerful new technology that is defining the role of individual genes in normal development, disease, and aging. In 2007, Evans shared the Nobel Prize in Physiology or Medicine with scientists Capecchi and Smithies for their discovery of "principles for introducing specific gene modifications in mice by the use of embryonic stem cells."

In the late 1980s, embryonic cells derived from primates were used to further develop ES cell culture technology. This led in 1998 to the first successful isolation and cultivation of human embryonic stem cells by James Thomson at the University of Wisconsin and John Gearhart at Johns Hopkins. Thomson used the inner cells from "leftover" donated in vitro fertilization (IVF) clinic blastocysts, whereas Gearhart worked with aborted fetal tissue.

Medical use of ES cells generated considerable controversy because it involved the destruction of a human embryo. In the United States from 2001 to 2009, these ethical concerns led to restriction of federal funds for human embryonic stem cell research. The issue was circumvented when Japanese geneticist Shinya Yamanaka in 2007 introduced a groundbreaking method to convert skin cells into analogues of stem cells. It had long been thought that cell specialization was irreversible, but Yamanaka demonstrated that with the insertion of a few genes, mature cells could be reprogrammed to become pluripotent, immature stem cells. Recent research has shown that these genetically repro-grammed or "induced" pluripotent stem cells (iPS cells) can give rise to all the different cell types of the body. They can be prepared from adult human cells, thus obviating the need for human embryonic tissue.

The proof that mature cells had all the genetic information needed for devel-opment of the adult organism was already brought by British scientist John Gurdon decades earlier. In 1958 Gurdon had replaced the immature cell nucleus of a frog's egg with that of a mature intestinal cell; his modified egg developed into a normal tadpole. The intense research generated by Gurdon's landmark discovery eventually led to the cloning of mammals. Yamanaka and Gurdon shared the 2012 Nobel Prize in Physiology or Medicine for discovering "that mature cells can be reprogrammed to become pluripotent."

Stem cell science has provided new tools to cure disease. Much of the interest in stem cell therapy has been driven by the shortage of donor organs for transplants. But the capacity of pluripotential stem cells to replicate and dif-ferentiate into specialized cells has also stimulated research in many other directions. Stem cells may be able to replace the function of myocardial cells killed by ischemic injury in heart attacks, pancreatic islets destroyed through autoimmune reactions in diabetes, or dopamine-producing neurons lost in Parkinson's disease.

The full potential of new stem cell therapies, regenerative medicine, and tissue engineering is yet to be realized. But the many recent innovations in biomedi-cine may well lead to viable therapeutic alternatives for conditions currently not amenable to conventional surgery or transplants. In 2008, a tracheal implant engi-neered with autologous stem cells successfully replaced an airway destroyed by tuberculosis. In 2010, a first therapeutic trial used human ES cells for patients with spinal injury. Stem cells also show great promise for the treatment of reti-nitis pigmentosa and age-related macular degeneration, two leading causes of blindness.

Tissue Engineering

In 2008 the first bioengineered airway was successfully transplanted into a 30-year-old Spanish mother of two with severe tuberculosis. Her infec-tion had led to the obstruction of a main bronchus and collapse of her left lung; she had been unable to carry out normal everyday tasks and was slowly dying. The new trachea provided her with a normally functioning airway and saved her life.

The 6.5-cm segment used for constructing the implant came from a 51-year-old donor who had died of cerebral hemorrhage. Using a technique developed at Padua University in Italy, the trachea was decellularized over a several-week period so that no donor cells remained to induce graft rejection. It took 25 cycles of rinsing to eliminate all donor antigens.

Meanwhile, at the University of Bristol, tissue-engineering teams led by ear/nose/throat (ENT) surgeon Martin Birchall and rheumatologist Anthony Hollander grew cultures of epithelial cells and stem cells taken from the recipient's own trachea and bone marrow. The bone marrow stem cells were differentiated and matured into cartilage cells (chondrocytes) using a method Hollander had devised to treat osteoarthritis. The outer scaffold of the donor's tracheal tube was then repopulated with these chondrocytes using a specially manufactured cell incubator (bioreactor) that allowed them to migrate into the tissue under ideal conditions. With the same method, epithelial cells were seeded onto the inside to replicate the inner lining of the trachea.

Four days after seeding, the hybrid graft was flown to Barcelona where it was inserted in place of the patient's damaged trachea by thoracic surgeon Paolo Macchiarini and his team. The patient did not develop antibodies to her graft and took no immunosuppressive drugs. Just a few days after transplantation, the graft was nearly indistinguishable from adjacent bronchial tissue. A month later, a biopsy elicited localized bleeding, showing that new blood vessels had already developed. Lung function tests performed two months after the operation were all in the high-normal range for a young woman. Five years later, the patient was reported to live normally, without complications, immunosuppressive medicines, or rejection of the implanted airway.

Surgical skill, technological innovation, and scientific vision together with an extraordinary international team effort led to this remarkable outcome: the restoration of normal breathing through an artificial windpipe engineered with the patient's own stem cells.

Sources: Macchiarini, Paolo, et al., "Clinical Transplantation of a Tissue-engineered Airway," *The Lancet* December 2008, 372 (9655): 2023–2030.

The Guardian, "A Revolution in Surgery," http://www.theguardian.com/society/video/2008/nov/19/claudia-castillo-trachea-transplant-surgery.

Ultimately, the hope is that stem cell–based therapy will do away with the need for human organ donation, allograft transplants, and lifelong immuno-suppression. Instead, it will aim to restore the function of diseased tissues and organs with regenerated, bioengineered, and stem cell–populated substitutes.

Bibliography and Suggested Readings

Bongso, Ariff, and Lee, Eng Hin, eds., *Stem Cells: From Bench to Bedside*, River Edge: World Scientific Publishing Co., 2005.

Little, Marie-Thérèse, and Storb, Rainer, "History of Haematopoietic Stem-Cell Transplantation," *Nature Reviews Cancer* March 2002: 2, 231–238.

Mummery, Christine, Wilmut, Sir Ian, van de Stolpe, Anja, and Roelen, Bernard, *Stem Cells: Scientific Facts and Fiction*, London: Academic Publishing, 2010.

Parson, Ann, *Proteus Effect: Stem Cells and Their Promise*, Washington, DC: Joseph Henry Press, 2004.

Solter, Davor, "From Teratocarcinomas to Embryonic Stem Cells and Beyond: A History of Embryonic Stem Cell Research," *Nature Reviews Genetics* April 2006: 7, 319–327.

Steinhoff, Gustav, ed., *Regenerative Medicine: From Protocol to Patient*, Dordrecht: Springer, 2013.

Thompson, Gilbert, ed., *Pioneers of Medicine without a Nobel Prize*, London: World Scientific Publishing, 2014.

Tests and Tools

Angiocardiography

What	Insertion of a flexible tube into the chambers of the heart through a peripheral vein or artery for diagnostic or therapeutic purposes.
Where	Germany; United States
When	1929; 1940
By Whom	Werner Forssmann (1904–1979); André Cournand (1895–1959); Dickinson Richards (1895–1973)
Importance	Key advance making possible detailed study of cardiac function; has become a standard diagnostic method for evaluating major cardiac diseases and is often mandatory prior to invasive therapy; laid the groundwork for interventional cardiology and treatment of coronary artery and other heart diseases by percutaneous routes.

The advent of cardiac catheterization revolutionized the field of cardiology and the diagnosis of coronary, valvular, and congenital heart disease. The technique, in which a thin, flexible catheter is threaded under fluoroscopic guidance from a peripheral blood vessel into the heart, has today become commonplace. Diagnostic catheterizations exceed 2,000,000 per year; in the Unites States alone, in 2010, 1 million were performed. Catheterization of the left heart via one of the femoral or radial arteries is used to diagnose coronary or valvular heart disease. The procedure usually includes imaging of the left ventricle and of the coronary vasculature, as well as measurement of left ventricular pressure. Right heart catheterization assesses function of the right heart and the pulmonary circulation. It measures oxygen saturations, pulmonary artery pressure, filling pressures, cardiac output, and more. Combined right and left catheterization helps evaluate complex cardiac conditions, including congenital disease or heart failure.

Physicians since Hippocratic times had used cadavers and experimental animals to study the heart and its function. In 1844 French physiologist Claude

Bernard described right and left heart catheterization by the femoral routes in a horse and a dog, recording intracardiac pressures and temperatures; he was the first to name the procedure. Jean-Baptiste Chauveau and Etienne Marey in France continued Bernard's research. They inserted a double-lumen catheter into a horse's heart to measure pressures and apical impulse and proved that systole was a dynamic process resulting from contraction of the heart muscle.

X-rays, fluoroscopy, and early arteriography with various contrast media were important late-19th-century advances crucial to the development of invasive cardiology in man. As late as the 1920s, however, many still considered that manipulating the living human heart was off-limits. Not only was it physically difficult to access and dangerous to the patient, but for many it meant invading the body's sacred, spiritual center.

A daring self-experiment performed in 1929 by 25-year-old German medical graduate Werner Forssmann changed the field. Forssmann, a surgical intern at a small hospital near Berlin, had become interested in cardiac arrest and was trying to develop an emergency technique for direct delivery of drugs into the heart for the purpose of resuscitation. This, he hypothesized, could be accomplished much more effectively via direct venous access to the right heart rather than through risky intracardiac injection. To test his theory, he inserted a 65-cm-long ureteric catheter into his left forearm and advanced the tip of the catheter through his cephalic vein "without resistance." He reported feeling slight warmth but no pain. With the help of a surgical nurse he then walked to the X-ray department and stood behind a fluoroscopic screen, while the nurse held up a mirror for him to see the position of the catheter. After pushing the tube into his right atrium he had an X-ray taken to document the position of the catheter inside the heart.

Forssmann was lucky. He suffered only a minor wound infection at the site of the incision in his arm. But his self-experiment caused a sensation. When he first published his account of the procedure his superiors were aghast, for it was widely held that any such invasion of the heart would be fatal. He was fired from an unpaid teaching post at Berlin's Charité Hospital and told he might lecture in a circus but not at a respectable German university. Over the next two years he continued animal experiments and injected various radio-opaque chemicals into his own heart to visualize the cardiac movements. Eventually, in the face of continued hostility from the medical establishment, reportedly after having used all his veins with multiple cut-downs, he gave up. In the mid-1930s he turned to a career in general surgery and urology.

Until Forssmann's experiment there had been little invasive study of the living human heart. Disease diagnosis relied on physical examination and use of the stethoscope, electrocardiography, and X-ray. A few early 20th-century studies with central drug injection and contrast angiography had been either unsuccessful or poorly documented. Contrast agent toxicity was another frequent problem. Still, the potential of Forssmann's technique as a diagnostic tool was quickly recognized. Between 1930 and 1940 researchers on both sides of the Atlantic contributed to its development, performing cardiac output studies and angiocardiograms. In 1941, using Forssmann's early method, André Cournand and Dickinson Richards in New York published their landmark investigations of right heart physiology in human patients, demonstrating that cardiac catheterization was safe. They had begun studying patients and healthy volunteers in 1936, after initial cadaver and dog experiments. They developed methods for right atrial blood sampling and demonstrated that catheters could be left in place for up to an hour without complications.

Cournand and Richards studied more than a hundred patients over the course of three years elucidating pathophysiological changes in various heart and lung diseases. They calculated cardiac output, confirming the principle developed by German physiologist Adolf Fick. They described the complex pressure–flow relation between the pulmonary circulation and the respiratory cycle and showed how chronic pulmonary disease affects not only the lungs but also the heart. They also defined the pathophysiology of cardiovascular shock, a major focus of investigation during World War II and shed light on circulatory failure as a result of blood loss or insufficient vascular tone. They showed the importance of right atrial filling pressure in maintaining cardiac output and the near-linear relationship between cardiac output and blood volume. They also demonstrated how vasoconstriction and fall in arterial pressure following blood loss reduced blood flow to many organs and how extracellular fluid shifts into the vascular space. Their findings represented new knowledge and still guide modern-day management of circulatory shock.

A flood of subsequent research followed this groundbreaking work. Lewis Dexter, Richard Bing, and James Warren carried out important studies on congenital heart disease. Dexter in Boston and Lars Werko in Sweden established that pulmonary capillary wedge pressure—gauged by wedging a catheter into a branch of the pulmonary artery—closely reflects left atrial pressure. Wedge pressure measurement with balloon-tipped, flow-directed catheters devised in 1970 by New York cardiologists Jeremy Swan and William Ganz revolutionized coronary care. It allowed pulmonary artery catheterization without fluoroscopy and made possible bedside hemodynamic monitoring, a critical tool in the care of surgical and cardiac patients.

In 1956, the Nobel Prize in Physiology or Medicine was awarded jointly to André Cournand, Werner Forssmann, and Dickinson Richards "for their discoveries concerning heart catheterization and pathological changes in the circulatory system." Forssmann, whose claim to precedence Cournand had acknowledged in the first sentence of his 1941 report, was "plucked from obscurity," unaware until a few years before that his work had not been forgotten.

Right heart catheterization, now considered safe, made investigation of cardiac and pulmonary function possible in many clinical situations. Accessing the left heart presented greater difficulties. Here the catheter must move against arterial flow and potential vasospasm, which could impede its progress; also, it can be moved into the left ventricle only during the brief time window in which the aortic valve leaflets are open. Early techniques to enter the left heart had included suprasternal and trans-septal left atrial puncture. By 1950, Cleveland cardiologist Henry Zimmerman reported the first retrograde left heart catheterizations via ulnar artery cut-down, crossing the aortic valve and entering the left ventricle in 11 patients with aortic insufficiency; a 12th patient died of ventricular fibrillation.

In 1953, Swedish physician Sven-Ivar Seldinger developed a safer percutaneous technique for introducing catheters using a sheath and a guidewire. Today, the Seldinger technique is used not only for right and left heart procedures, but also for inserting chest tubes, central venous lines, leads for pacemakers and implantable cardiac defibrillators, and many other interventional procedures.

Until 1958, no one had succeeded in effective imaging of the coronary circulation. It was then, during an aortographic procedure, that Cleveland cardiologist Mason Sones inadvertently injected contrast dye into a patient's right coronary, in effect obtaining the first selective coronary angiogram. Sones's method was a watershed in modern cardiology: it provided the first detailed images of coronary obstructions. Refined in 1967 by Melvin Judkins and Kurt Amplatz, and more recently by Montreal cardiologist Lucien Campeau who introduced a safer radial artery approach, it ultimately led to the now widely employed coronary angiography. This remains the gold standard for evaluation of ischemic heart disease.

Cardiac catheterization has allowed clinicians to gain the in-depth understanding of cardiac and circulatory physiology without which coronary surgery and catheter-based interventions such as angioplasty would have been impossible. Today the technique guides the care of millions of acute and chronic cardiac patients. The 1956 Nobel Committee paid tribute to Forssmann's conviction in the pursuit of his research, despite the prejudice that ultimately deflected his course and hampered earlier exploitation of his ideas. Forssmann's courageous self-experiment changed the science and practice of medicine.

Bibliography and Suggested Readings

Altman, Lawrence K., *Who Goes First? The Story of Self-Experimentation in Medicine*, Berkeley: University of California Press, 1998.

Baim, Donald S., ed., *Grossman's Cardiac Catheterization, Angiography, and Intervention,* 7th ed., Philadelphia: Lippincott, Williams & Wilkins, 2006.

Centers for Disease Control and Prevention, 2016, "Inpatient Surgery," http://www.cdc.gov/nchs/fastats/inpatient-surgery.htm.

Cournand Andre, and Ranges, Hilmert A., "Catheterization of the Right Auricle in Man," *Proceedings of the Society for Experimental Biology and Medicine* 1941, 46: 462.

Forssmann-Falck, Renate, "Werner Forssmann: A Pioneer of Cardiology," *American Journal of Cardiology*, March 1997, 79(5): 651–660.

Mueller, Richard L., and Sanborn, Timothy A., "The History of Interventional Cardiology: Cardiac Catheterization, Angioplasty, and Related Interventions," *American Heart Journal* 1995, 129: 146–172.

"The Nobel Prize in Physiology or Medicine 1956," 2016, http://www.nobelprize.org/nobel_prizes/medicine/laureates/1956.

Seed, Tony, "The Introduction of Cardiac Catheterization," in Thompson, Gilbert, *Nobel Prizes That Changed Medicine.* Singapore: World Scientific Publishing Co., 2011: 69–87.

Zimmerman, Henry A., et al., "Catheterization of the Left Side of the Heart in Man," *Circulation* 1950, 1: 357–359.

Clinical Trials

What	Biomedical or behavioral research study of human subjects designed to determine, through the use of objective mathematical and statistical methods, the benefits of new medical treatments or of new tests for prevention, screening, and diagnosis.
Where	United Kingdom; France; United States
When	1830s; 1940s
By Whom	Pierre Louis (1787–1872); Ronald Fisher (1890–1962); Austin Bradford Hill (1897–1991); Archibald Cochrane (1909–1988)
Importance	Helps define the efficacy and safety of new drugs or treatments, thus supporting rational therapies.

Clinical trials are experiments in which participants are assigned to study groups, one experimental and the other(s) serving as a comparison or control group. Subjects in the experimental group are treated with the drug under investigation, whereas the control group is given either a known treatment or a "placebo," a nonactive substance such as a sugar pill. Subject randomization aims to control for variables other than the drug or therapy being studied. Additional measures to eliminate potential bias include masking or "blinding": in single-blind studies, the subjects do not know which group they have been assigned to; in double-blind studies, neither the subjects nor the investigators know the specific assignments. To be statistically meaningful, results require a sufficiently large number of study participants.

Historically, physicians had long compared treated and untreated patients to evaluate the benefit of new therapies, but such reports usually consisted only of individual case histories. The first clinical studies involving elementary quantitative analysis were reported in the 1700s when British physician James Jurin, an early advocate of smallpox inoculation, compared the death rates of cases of naturally contracted smallpox to those occurring after inoculation. His 1723 *Account of the Success of Inoculating the Small-Pox* demonstrated the efficacy of the new practice. Another example is the famous 1747 study of naval surgeon James Lind who studied the effects of diet in 12 sailors afflicted by scurvy, "their cases as similar as I could have them." He found the "most sudden and visible good effects were perceived from the use of the oranges and lemons." Lind's small sample was not statistically significant, yet it provided an effective rationale for the use of citrus fruit to prevent scurvy.

The development of statistical methods in the early 19th century led to the use of mortality tables and related data as an index of community health. In clinical medicine, the work of French physician-pathologist Pierre C. A. Louis was seminal in furthering this numerical approach. To preclude bias and draw valid conclusions, Louis advocated collecting observations on large numbers of patients and comparing treatments in "indiscriminately" chosen cases "of as similar a description as you could find . . ." His "méthode numérique" is considered the forerunner to modern clinical trials and influenced future practitioners on both sides of the Atlantic.

The work of 19th-century physiologists such as Claude Bernard further encouraged application of experimental methods to clinical medicine. At the same time, growing numbers of patients in the great city hospitals made for readily available subjects for statistical comparison. Ignaz Semmelweis, who established the importance of hand washing in preventing the spread of childbed fever, had based his conclusions on the highly disparate mortality statistics he observed in two separate maternity wards within the same hospital. Suspecting that infections were due to "the conveyance . . . of putrid particles . . . through the agency of the examining fingers," he required all students and physicians to scrub their hands with chlorinated lime. This simple practice resulted in a significant decrease in postpartum fatalities. Joseph Lister used similar comparative statistics to evaluate the effects of his antiseptic technique on mortality following surgical amputations.

Investigation of nutritional diseases such as Goldberger's classic 1914 study of pellagra became another important area for the development of clinical trials. However, most early studies validated preventive methods, not therapeutic interventions. For the increasingly plentiful drugs and patent medicines available on the marketplace there was no mechanism in place to test efficacy or safety. By the early 20th century, the proliferation of pharmaceuticals of all sorts led to efforts to assess their manufacturers' claims. In the United States, they included the establishment of the Council on Pharmacy and Chemistry by the American Medical Association and the 1906 passage of the Pure Food and Drug Act. But attempts to evaluate treatments encountered various difficulties, including failure to standardize methods and protocols, controversies among investigators, and lack of resources. Patient variability also came into play, as did the often well-founded preferences and biases of individual practitioners. All these factors affected trial results, making them difficult to reproduce or to use as a foundation for therapeutic guidelines.

At the request of the Association of British Chemical Manufacturers, the British Medical Research Council (MRC) in 1931 formed a Therapeutic Trials Committee in order to evaluate new drugs. Its task was to develop testing standards and provide impartial clinical reports on new drugs to be placed on the market. The committee applied alternate selection methods early on in recruiting control subjects so as to ensure comparability of experimental groups and to eliminate investigator bias.

By 1940, the problem of clinical experimentation had been well defined. The work of English biologist R. A. Fisher, who pioneered many of the principles of experimental design and data analysis, supported the use of strict randomization. Scarce resources and rationing of new medicines, especially antibiotics, during and after World War II also fostered the adoption of the concept of standardized, statistically based protocols.

The British Medical Research Council, from 1946 to 1948, was first to conduct a statistically valid clinical trial with properly randomized control subjects. The MRC trial, carefully planned and executed under the direction of statistician Austin Bradford Hill, was both double blind and placebo controlled; it was designed to test the new antibiotic streptomycin in the treatment of pulmonary tuberculosis. Its 107 patients were accrued from several centers and randomly allocated to treatment or nontreatment groups through a system of sealed envelopes. These trials were the only way most British patients could receive the rationed drug. The *British Medical Journal* noted that randomization "removed personal responsibility from the clinician" for selecting which patients might benefit from the new treatment.

To ensure objective assessment, two radiologists and one clinician interpreted patient X-rays, each working independently and without knowledge of group assignments. This blinded protocol, together with a statistically based study design, strengthened end-point evaluation and validated the eventual conclusions: both patient survival and radiological findings were significantly improved on streptomycin.

Austin Bradford Hill was instrumental in the subsequent development of controlled clinical trials. His writings defined many fundamental issues, such as eligibility of patients, concurrent controls, random allocation, and statistical analysis. Hill was a major contributor to later trials in rheumatoid arthritis and cerebrovascular disease and to field trials of various vaccines. Together with epidemiologist Richard Doll, he also carried out landmark studies on the correlation between lung cancer and smoking, including the long-term prospective "British Doctors' Study."

The massive polio vaccine trials of 1954 most clearly demonstrated the usefulness of randomized controlled trials (RCTs). They showed that rigorous experimental methods could demonstrate the validity of therapeutic and prophylactic innovations, and contributed to establishing the authority of clinical trials within the international medical community.

Nevertheless, it took some years before randomization was accepted as a normal procedure. The chemotherapeutic revolution of the 1950s introduced hundreds of new drugs every year. Pharmaceutical companies seeking to establish their products increasingly sponsored clinical trials. Not all of them met scientific standards; even the *Journal of the American Medical Association* warned that "[use of] the double-blind technique . . . [could] not validate otherwise poorly designed experiments." In the United States, the Food and Drug Administration (FDA) had the authority to scrutinize new drugs. In the summer of 1962, reports of the severe malformations caused by pregnant women's use of the drug thalidomide led to the enactment of the Kefauver-Harris Amendments, which gave the FDA even greater powers. In 1970, the FDA called for "adequate and well-controlled investigations" in the form of clinical trials using a statistical, scientific model to regulate the drug industry. As a result, the pharmaceutical industry adapted their resource allocations to meet these requirements.

Increasing recognition of RCTs spawned the movement of "evidence-based medicine" (EBM), a term coined at Canadian McMaster University. Scottish epidemiologist Archibald Cochrane was an early proponent, advocating

The Nuremberg Code

The Nuremberg Code was developed after the "Doctors' Trial" (**United States of America v. Karl Brandt, et al.**) in 1947, the first of twelve trials for Nazi war crimes held in Nuremberg after World War II. A landmark document governing research and experimentation on human subjects, the code lists major ethical principles such as informed consent and beneficence. It has been further elaborated in the 1964 Declaration of Helsinki and its later revisions.

The tenets of the Nuremberg Code are:

1. The voluntary consent of the human subject is absolutely essential.

   This means that the person involved should have legal capacity to give consent; should be so situated as to be able to exercise free power of choice, without the intervention of any element of force, fraud, deceit, duress, over-reaching, or other ulterior form of constraint or coercion; and should have sufficient knowledge and comprehension of the elements of the subject matter involved, as to enable him to make an understanding and enlightened decision. This latter element requires that, before the acceptance of an affirmative decision by the experimental subject, there should be made known to him the nature, duration, and purpose of the experiment; the method and means by which it is to be conducted; all inconveniences and hazards reasonably to be expected; and the effects upon his health or person, which may possibly come from his participation in the experiment.

   The duty and responsibility for ascertaining the quality of the consent rests upon each individual who initiates, directs or engages in the experiment. It is a personal duty and responsibility, which may not be delegated to another with impunity.

2. The experiment should be such as to yield fruitful results for the good of society, unprocurable by other methods or means of study, and not random and unnecessary in nature.

3. The experiment should be so designed and based on the results of animal experimentation and a knowledge of the natural history of the disease or other problem under study, that the anticipated results will justify the performance of the experiment.

4. The experiment should be so conducted as to avoid all unnecessary physical and mental suffering and injury.

5. No experiment should be conducted, where there is an *a priori* reason to believe that death or disabling injury will occur; except, perhaps, in those experiments where the experimental physicians also serve as subjects.

6. The degree of risk to be taken should never exceed that determined by the humanitarian importance of the problem to be solved by the experiment.

7. Proper preparations should be made and adequate facilities provided to protect the experimental subject against even remote possibilities of injury, disability, or death.

8. The experiment should be conducted only by scientifically qualified persons . . .

9. During the course of the experiment, the human subject should be at liberty to bring the experiment to an end, if he has reached the physical or mental state, where continuation of the experiment seemed to him to be impossible.

10. During the course of the experiment, the scientist in charge must be prepared to terminate the experiment at any stage, if he has probable cause to believe . . . that a continuation of the experiment is likely to result in injury, disability, or death to the experimental subject.

Source: "Trials of War Criminals before the Nuremberg Military Tribunals under Control Council Law No. 10," Vol. 2, pp. 181–182. Washington, DC: U.S. Government Printing Office, 1949.

systematic analysis and meta-analysis of the accumulating mass of clinical trial data in order to establish definitive benefits and to improve therapeutic practices.

In the 21st century, randomized controlled trials have become an essential component of medical research. Hailed as a major, scientifically sound innovation, they are widely accepted as the "gold standard" for establishing therapeutic efficacy of new medicines and medical techniques. They are subject to regulatory ethical scrutiny, but underscore the value of clinical experimentation on human subjects to deliver objective data on the efficacy and safety of medicines, and to aid clinicians in making treatment decisions.

Bibliography and Suggested Readings

Gallin, John I., and Ognibene, Frederick, eds., *Principles and Practice of Clinical Research,* 2nd ed., Burlington: Academic Press, 2007.

Keating, Peter, and Cambrosio, Alberto, "Cancer Clinical Trials: The Emergence and Development of a New Style of Practice," *Bulletin of the History of Medicine* 2007, 81(1): 197–223.

Lederer, Susan, *Subjected to Science: Human Experimentation in America before the Second World War,* Baltimore: Johns Hopkins University Press, 1995.

Lilienfeld, A., "The Fielding H. Garrison Lecture: Ceteris Paribus: The Evolution of the Clinical Trial," *Bulletin of the History of Medicine* 1982, 56(1): 1–18.

Mann, John, *Life Saving Drugs: The Elusive Magic Bullet,* Cambridge: Royal Society of Chemistry, 2004.

Marks, Harry M., *The Progress of Experiment: Science and Therapeutic Reform in the United States, 1900–1990,* Cambridge, New York: Cambridge University Press, 1997.

Meldrum, Marcia, "A Brief History of the Randomized Controlled Trial: From Oranges and Lemons to the Gold Standard," *Hematology/Oncology Clinics of North America* August 1, 2000, 14(4): 745–760.

Pocock, Stuart J., *Clinical Trials: A Practical Approach,* Somerset: Wiley, 2013.

Valier, H., and Timmermann, C., "Clinical Trials and the Reorganization of Medical Research in Post-Second World War Britain," *Medical History* 2008, 52(4): 493–510.

Computed Tomography (CT)

What	Computed tomography (CT), also computed axial tomography or computer assisted tomography (CAT), is a technique that uses X-ray technology to produce cross-sectional, tomographic (the term is derived from the Greek *tomos*, "slice", and *graphein*, "write") images of specific areas of the body for diagnostic purposes.
Where	England; South Africa; United States
When	1963; 1967
By Whom	Godfrey Newbold Hounsfield (1919–2004); Allen McLeod Cormack (1924–1998)
Importance	Major advance in diagnostic radiology providing accurate non-invasive data; more precise than X-ray imaging, permitting visualization without inference and thus more accurate diagnostic information.

Computed tomography scanning uses X-rays to produce a series of computer-processed cross-sectional images that result in a detailed three-dimensional representation. Different image shades are due to differential absorption, with denser tissues absorbing more of the X-ray beam. Whereas standard X-rays project superimposed shadows of different structures, CT scanning eliminates this superimposition so that there are no overlapping image elements. In addition, sensitive crystal detectors, together with signal amplification, allow exceptionally high resolution of different densities, making possible a precise image of a thin slice of the body and of individual organs.

Since its discovery in 1967, computed tomography has become a core constituent of medical diagnostic imaging. The first commercial CT scanner was the work of Sir Godfrey Hounsfield, an informally trained British engineer who became an expert in radar technology while in the Royal Air Force. Hounsfield had been investigating the problems of pattern recognition at EMI (Electric and Music Industries) Central Research Laboratories when he considered assembling a three-dimensional representation of the contents of a box from a set of readings taken through the object at randomly selected directions. He found that this could be accomplished by shining X-ray beams from different directions and then reconstructing the three-dimensional object as a series of slices, using computers to analyze the vast amount of data.

Hounsfield soon started looking for practical applications and in 1968 patented his technique as a "method of and apparatus for examination of the body by radiation . . ." He succeeded in enlisting the support of the Department of Health and Social Security (DHSS) by presenting his proposed machine as an opportunity to visualize the brain. Such a device would not only be cost effective for cerebral disorders that often required exploratory surgery, but the promise of insight into the brain which, since the beginning of X-ray diagnosis, had remained a challenge, stirred popular imagination. DHSS agreed to support Hounsfield's research, deciding to develop a machine intended for neuroradiologists that would scan the head.

The first prototype EMI brain scanner was installed in Atkinson Morley's Hospital at Wimbledon. Scanning time was four minutes per slice, each approximately 1 cm thick. The computer was separate from the scanner, so that imaging data had to be recorded on magnetic tape and transported to the EMI laboratories for analysis. The first patient scanned was a 41-year-old woman with symptoms of frontal lobe disease. Her scan, during which she had to lie with her head propped against a water-filled box (this reduced the amount of X-ray data to be processed), took 15 hours to complete! The cross-sectional image ultimately obtained revealed a circular cyst in the patient's left frontal lobe. It was subsequently excised, and James Ambrose, the neurosurgeon in charge who

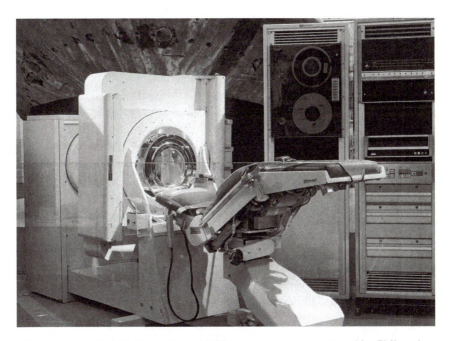

Early model of Sir Godfrey Hounsfield's brain scanner produced by EMI in the early 1970s. CT (computerized tomography) rapidly became a key diagnostic modality, particularly for imaging of the brain. CT scanning constructs cross-sectional images of body "slices," using a computer program to analyze data derived from a series of precision X-ray exposures. Today, tens of millions of scans are performed every year for diagnostic and screening purposes. (Science & Society Picture Library/Getty Images)

himself had been investigating alternative cranial imaging techniques, became a key figure in the early development of CT scanning and neuroradiology.

Ambrose and Hounsfield presented their sensational findings at the annual meeting of the British Institute of Radiology in April 1972 in a paper entitled "Computerized Axial Tomography (A New Means of Demonstrating Some of the Soft Tissues of the Brain Without the Use of Contrast Media)." Additional publications later that year described Hounsfield's theories and techniques and Ambrose's clinical findings; a third paper considered the important, and still debated, issue of radiation doses. In 1973 Hounsfield summarized the new scanning system as "a technique in which X-ray transmission readings are taken through the head at a multitude of angles: from these data, absorption values of the material contained within the head are calculated on a computer and presented as a series of pictures of slices of the cranium. The system is approximately 100 times more sensitive than conventional X-ray systems to such an extent that variations in soft tissues of nearly similar density can be displayed."

How to produce a three-dimensional image of an interior slice of an object by reconstructing information obtained from multiple projections through the object had been a subject of research since the 1930s. South African physicist Allen Cormack had developed its theoretical mathematics while monitoring radiation therapy at Groote Schuur Hospital in Cape Town. Realizing that treatment planning could be vastly improved if the absorption coefficients of different organs could be determined, he set out to find a way to map heterogeneous body tissues and densities using X-rays. He was unaware of Austrian mathematician Johann Radon's 1917 solution to the problem: his *Radon transform* demonstrated that if line integrals of an object's density are known for all lines intersecting a slice of this object, then its density can be reconstructed. This formula was applicable to the creation of an image by radiation scattering data associated with cross-sectional scans.

Cormack published his work in 1964, but there was little commercial interest in his publication. Reportedly, the Swiss Center for Avalanche Research expressed interest: indeed, his method could be applied to measure density of snow on a mountain. Cormack was the first to state the principles for reconstructing a cross-section of organ tissues based on x-ray projections, anticipating the development of computer-assisted tomography by several years. Presumably the reason his discovery was not industrially applied at the time was that contemporary computer technology lacked sufficient capacity.

In 1979, Hounsfield and Cormack were awarded the Nobel Prize in Physiology or Medicine, a confirmation of the value of their technique. The new CT scanning technology marked a turning point in the history of traditional diagnostic radiology. It revolutionized the imaging of the nervous system, finally making possible the visualization of the brain and replacing invasive pneumoencephalography procedures, where air was injected into the cerebrospinal fluid to delineate brain masses or abnormal ventricles. Hounsfield's system, first directed at the examination of the brain, was rapidly expanded to whole-body scanning.

Initially the expense of the new technique limited its use. Within a few years, however, the early apparatus passed through several generations and was increasingly manufactured by a number of industrial companies. Later technical improvements including 3D and helical scanning; rapid analytical computer reconstruction methods improved performance and quality. As a result, time for data acquisition was significantly reduced. Nowadays, although radiation exposure remains a concern, scanning takes only seconds.

Computed tomography changed the way radiologists look at the body. In medicine it transformed clinical care, and in radiotherapy it helped define diseased areas to be irradiated. CT is especially useful in critical care settings, where it aids in acute diagnoses such as intracranial hemorrhage, trauma, and stroke.

Bibliography and Suggested Readings

Gunderman, Richard B., *X-Ray Vision: The Evolution of Medical Imaging and Its Human Significance*, Oxford: Oxford University Press, 2013.

Hounsfield, Godfrey, "Computerized Transverse Axial Scanning (Tomography): Part 1, Description of System," *British Journal of Radiology* 1973, 46: 1016–1022.

Kevles, Bettyann H., *Naked to the Bone: Medical Imaging in the Twentieth Century*, New Brunswick: Rutgers University Press, 1997.

Thomas, Adrian M. K., and Banerjee, Arpan K., *History of Radiology*, Oxford: Oxford University Press, 2013.

Electrocardiogram (ECG)

What	A visual tracing of the electrical activity and conduction system of the heart over time, measured by electrodes affixed to the skin, and displayed by a specialized external device.
Where	Leiden, Holland
When	1903
By Whom	Willem Einthoven (1860–1927)
Importance	Provides best objective technique to record the heartbeat and to evaluate cardiac function; indispensable for diagnosing heart disease and monitoring treatment effectiveness; essential tool in screening and risk stratification in athletes and prevention of sudden death.

The discovery of the electrocardiogram (ECG or EKG) at the turn of the 19th century ushered in a new era in the diagnosis and treatment of heart disease. Several decades earlier the introduction of the stethoscope had led to a rapid expansion of cardiovascular science. It was soon learned that the cyclic contractions of the heart muscle, which produce the energy to propel blood through the circulatory system, were accompanied by electric activity. This electrical current, or action potential, measured in only millivolts, is reflected at the body surface in the very weak electrical potential fluctuations that accompany the heartbeat.

Until the discovery of electrocardiography, diagnosis of heart disorders was made primarily through physical examination; additional techniques employed were polygraphic recordings of vascular pulsations, or sphygmomanometry, to measure blood pressure. The electrocardiograph, however, could detect the minute electrical impulses generated by polarization and depolarization of the myocardial tissue and translate this information into specific waveforms by means of an electromechanical device. This instrument, a specialized galvanometer, deflected a pointer or needle attached to a moving coil in a magnetic field and recorded the resulting movement, itself proportional to the intensity of current passing through the coil. It thus provided much more specific information about the rhythm and mode of propagation of the cardiac impulse.

A first crude electrocardiogram was produced in 1887 by British physiologist Augustus Waller. Waller recorded the electrical activity of the heart muscle using surface electrodes and a capillary electrometer, a device developed to detect small bursts of electric current; he performed many of his experiments on his favorite bulldog, Jimmy, made to stand in pots of saline solution, which led to accusations of animal cruelty. Waller lectured widely on his technique but did not recognize its clinical potential.

It was Willem Einthoven, professor of physiology at the University of Leiden, who by means of a refined *string galvanometer* developed a very sensitive electrocardiograph. Inspired by Waller, Einthoven had begun to study myocardial action potentials first using a capillary electrometer. He then worked on improving this method in order to obtain higher-quality tracings. By 1902, Einthoven's instrument could translate the electrical activity of the heart into very specific, reproducible visual patterns, registering electric potential fluctuations of very high frequency and allowing both high sensitivity and short adjustment time. This initial electrocardiograph was a complex contraption, which conducted the electrical signals of the heart muscle through a silver-coated quartz fiber suspended in an electromagnetic field and deflected them at right angles to this field. A moving glass photographic plate recorded the fiber's shadow; this was what constituted the electrocardiographic tracing.

The first ECG recorded with the string galvanometer, published in 1903, was strikingly similar to modern tracings. It represented a distinct, directly readable image of the electrical impulses of the heart. Einthoven labeled the individual waves with the letters "PQRST," a notation based on mathematical conventions and still used in contemporary ECG interpretation.

Einthoven published his original paper on normal and abnormal ECGs in 1906, describing not only electrocardiographic features of a number of cardiac disorders, but also application of electrocardiography to clinical examination.

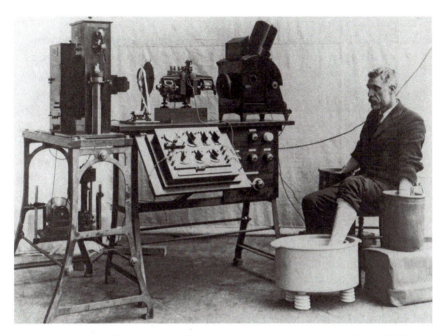

An early version of Einthoven's electrocardiograph machine, built ca. 1912 by the Cambridge Scientific Instrument Company. Before the advent of modern contact electrodes, the patient's hands and one foot were immersed in buckets of salt solution to conduct the electrical current from the skin to the apparatus, producing what is known as Einthoven's triangle. (FPB/Hulton Archive/Getty Images)

Clearly, he had recognized the diagnostic value of this new technique. In 1909 he published a detailed description of his instrument. The early machines were large and cumbersome and were mainly confined to laboratories or hospitals. They needed several technicians to operate and required study subjects to immerse their limbs in containers of saline solution, thus making the device impractical for routine clinical use.

Nonetheless, as the Nobel Committee later pointed out, it was clear that Einthoven's new method of investigation filled an important need in medicine. British cardiologist Thomas Lewis was among the first to recognize this and helped establish electrocardiography in clinical settings. In 1908, he demonstrated the role of Einthoven's discovery in the diagnosis of cardiac rhythm disorders, especially that of heart block. In 1913, he published the first treatise on the new technique, describing its medical applications. Meanwhile, in 1912, Chicago physician James Herrick defined the clinical features of coronary thrombosis and its associated electrocardiographic changes in a landmark article on myocardial infarction. In New York, Harold Pardee described the characteristic sequential ECG changes in acute myocardial infarction. Thus, in delineating objective signs of disease, electrocardiography was not only diagnostic but also prognostic. By 1930, the important role of the ECG in the diagnosis of myocardial infarction had been widely accepted; current data show that study of consecutive ECG tracings has a 95 percent diagnostic accuracy in the course of a myocardial infarction.

In the 1930s Michigan cardiologist Frank Wilson further advanced the new technology with his design of the modern-day unipolar chest leads, which allowed more sensitive recording in the frontal and precordial planes. In 1938, the American Heart Association and the British Cardiac Society recommended the present six precordial locations for the exploring electrode. Later, augmented unipolar limb leads were included in the 12-lead ECG currently in use.

Willem Einthoven was awarded the 1924 Nobel Prize in Physiology or Medicine "for his discovery of the mechanism of the electrocardiogram." His work was fundamental to the development of modern cardiology. Electrocardiography, together with other diagnostic technologies, became a symbol of the modern hospital and of modern medicine.

Electrocardiograms helped to visualize, measure, and identify a material basis for disease symptoms. ECG waves measured the rate and rhythm of the heart, derived its size and position, and indicated the presence of any damage. They also reflected the effects of drugs or therapeutic devices such as pacemakers. With the ECG, it became possible to diagnose multiple conditions, including ventricular hypertrophy (thickening of the ventricular walls), pericardial disease, life-threatening arrhythmias, and—last but not least—heart attacks and their warning signs. Electrocardiography thus became central to expanding clinical knowledge of heart disease. An objective screening tool, it also helped to establish norms for the healthy patient in routine examinations.

The new technology spawned multiple clinical applications. Exercise ECGs diagnose latent ischemic heart disease, and continuous recordings ("Holter" ECG) or electrophysiological studies can identify dangerous heart rhythms or conduction abnormalities. In the hospital setting, ECGs have become essential in monitoring the evolution of ischemic heart disease, watching metabolic disturbances, or assessing the success of electrical therapies such as cardioversion, pacemakers, and implantable defibrillators.

Over the years, technical advances reduced the weight and size of ECG machines. Most newer compact electronic devices use digital recording; often portable, they can be operated by a single technician. They allow for continuous heart monitoring and provide computerized interpretations of tracings. The form and quality of modern ECG tracings, however, are very much like Einthoven's early recordings. In a world where cardiovascular disease is one of the leading causes of mortality and morbidity, electrocardiography remains the gold standard for diagnosis to this day.

Bibliography and Suggested Readings

Bayés de Luna, Antoni, *Clinical Electrocardiography*, Oxford: Wiley-Blackwell, 2012.

Cooper, John K., "Electrocardiography 100 Years Ago. Origins, Pioneers, and Contributors," *New England Journal of Medicine* 1986, 315(7): 461–464.

Einthoven, Wilhelm, "The Different Forms of the Human Electrocardiogram and their Signification," *Lancet* 1912, 179(4622): 853–861.

Fisch, Charles. "Centennial of the String Galvanometer and the Electrocardiogram." *Journal of the American College of Cardiology* 2000, 36(6): 1737–1745.

Snellen, Herman A., *Willem Einthoven (1860–1927) Father of Electrocardiography: Life and Work, Ancestors and Contemporaries*, Dordrecht: Springer Netherlands, 1995.

Electroencephalogram (EEG)

What	Technology that visualizes brain activity through graphical recording of the electrical activity generated by cerebral neurons.
Where	Germany
When	1929
By Whom	Hans Berger (1873–1941)
Importance	Key diagnostic method in modern neuroscience; changed the understanding of epilepsies as neurologic conditions affecting electric signaling in the brain, rather than as psychiatric diseases.

Electroencephalography is a noninvasive technology used in evaluating psychiatric and neurological disorders. It records the spontaneous, intrinsic electrical activity of the brain over time by means of electrodes attached to the patient's scalp. The electrodes measure the voltage fluctuations reflecting movement of electrically charged ions across neuronal membranes. The recorded oscillations—the "brain waves"—are examined and interpreted according to standardized parameters and are an essential tool in differential diagnosis, especially when correlated with clinical manifestations.

British physiologist Richard Caton in 1875 was the first to document that the brain emitted electrical potentials. Using unipolar electrodes placed on the living, exposed brain of experimental animals, he registered superficial electrical impulses with a galvanometer. He detected clear alterations in brain electricity with various external stimuli; thus, the visual cortex of a dog generated large electrical potentials in response to light. He also found that current intensity increased during sleep and with impending death; after death, the currents disappeared. Others confirmed his findings. In 1891 Polish physiologist Adolf Beck showed that the brain had continuous low-level electrical activity peaking with sensory stimuli. This work anticipated the discovery of evoked nerve potentials in response to sensory stimuli in human subjects.

Human electroencephalography was the brainchild of German psychiatrist Hans Berger. In the early 1900s, technical improvements in radio signal amplifiers had made recording of electrical activity from the outer surface of the skull possible. Together with graphic methods of scientific analysis, this paved the way to investigating human subjects and psychic processes. Berger, who had a strong interest in psychophysiology and the relationship between mind and brain, believed in the theory of energy conservation in mind–brain interactions: energy generated to produce thought in one part of the brain must at the same time be dissipated in another part. Therefore, given precise measurements of metabolic energy—heat or electricity—in the cerebral cortex, it was theoretically possible to calculate equivalents of "psychic" energy: perception, feelings, conscious thought, and perhaps even mental telepathy.

Berger, familiar with the work of Italian physiologist Angelo Mosso, began studying changes in cerebral blood flow, the prime index of the amount of energy supplied to the brain. Like Mosso, he experimented using patients with surgical or traumatic skull defects that exposed their brains, measuring changes in cerebral blood flow in response to specific stimuli, and variations in cerebral temperature correlated to metabolic activity of the brain. None of these studies, however, captured meaningful information about energy transformation in the cerebral cortex.

In 1924, Berger tried recording electrical signals from the cortex of a 17-year-old patient who had undergone two craniostomies for the removal of a brain tumor. He soon discovered that these signals could also be detected on an intact skull and recorded the first human scalp EEG, using large electrodes positioned over the frontal and occipital areas. A diary entry reflected his trepidation at the prospect of fulfilling at last his long-held dream, the creation of a sort of "brain mirror."

Over the next five years, all the while refining his technical apparatus, he produced hundreds of EEGs of clinic patients, employees, himself, and his teenage son. He employed many of the same mental tasks he had used earlier and recorded EEGs of patients with brain tumors, dementia, epilepsy, and other neuropsychiatric conditions. After painstaking control studies, he finally published his findings in 1929, naming his technique "electroencephalography."

A series of landmark papers followed, in which Berger addressed the neurophysiological foundations and clinical applications of the EEG. He described two fundamental waveforms: the prominent alpha waves of longer duration correlated to mental activity, and the shorter beta waves were associated with cortical metabolism. He also demonstrated slowing of EEG response in hypoglycemic states, delirium, and other encephalopathies. His alpha and beta EEG wave components remain central to modern electroencephalography.

In the following decade neurologists and psychiatrists actively explored the potential use of the new technology. British electrophysiologist Edgar Douglas Adrian, whose work on neuronal function won him the 1932 Nobel Prize, was instrumental in further defining and establishing the validity of EEG results. His studies stimulated the use of electroencephalography as a scientific research tool in neuropsychiatry and brought international recognition to Berger's innovation.

In the United States neurologists William Lennox and Frederic Gibbs pioneered the use of EEG in investigating seizure disorders after learning that in experimental animals, administration of convulsive agents produced seizures accompanied by high-voltage brain impulses. Gibbs and his team characterized specific EEG patterns and waveforms, establishing their relationship to clinical states such as *petit mal* seizures, complex partial seizures, and other forms of epilepsy.

After World War II, the new technology expanded rapidly. Scientists began studying electrical activity of the brain both in psychiatric patients and in normal controls during various cognitive activities. EEG laboratories were established, technical improvements were made, and professional societies and journals founded. Experts increasingly regarded the EEG signal as a reliable scientific gauge of brain function.

Soon the new method was applied to an array of psychiatric, psychological, and psychophysiological phenomena. Psychologist Donald Lindsley, who became president of the American EEG Society, was among the first in his field to promote the use of electroencephalography for wide-ranging study of cerebral activities. His research defined the mechanisms of arousal and wakefulness and the role of the brainstem's reticular activating system. Until then, it had been accepted that wakefulness was only the result of afferent sensory stimulation of the cerebral cortex. Other researchers attempted to correlate brain waves and their variable oscillations with individual intelligence, emotion, or personality. Homosexuality, psychopathy, delinquency, and even peptic ulcer disease became the focus of EEG inquiry.

An early problem in EEG investigations was the interpretation and standardization of complex signals. Until the early 1960s, methodological criteria were lacking. Site-specific practices such as diverging electrode placement frequently accounted for diagnostic discrepancies. Initially, analysis relied only on visual inspection; for instance, sleep stages were determined by visual correlation of patterns of EEG activity and eye movements. Yet the significance of the waveforms generated by the brain was not obvious but had to be deciphered. An interpretative system had to be devised that would quantify rhythms and amplitudes and relate them to specific physiological conditions, giving meaning to the electrical signals.

Even so, capturing complex psychological processes remained elusive. In psychiatric patients, abnormalities in EEG tracings were minor and nonspecific, limiting the technique's usefulness for diagnosis. Of greatest utility were EEG findings in epilepsy and encephalopathy, for they most strongly correlated with clinical disease. EEG was also helpful in detecting structural, space-occupying brain lesions, themselves often associated with psychiatric symptoms: suspected brain tumors, stroke syndromes, and other disorders. Focal slowing of tracings could recognize 90 percent of tumors of the outer cortex.

Prior to the introduction of high-resolution neuroimaging, the discovery of electroencephalography was a milestone. EEG was a specific, noninvasive investigative tool at a time when the only available methods to detect and localize brain pathology were lumbar puncture and pneumoencephalography. Today EEG is used in neurological and neurosurgical practice for the diagnosis of epilepsies, sleep disorders, encephalopathies, coma, and confirmation of brain death.

The brain's cognitive functions—its processing and storage of information— continue to be the focus of active investigation in psychophysiology and experimental psychology. Since the 1960s and 1970s spectral signal analysis and advanced digital computers, which can rapidly process vast sets of multichannel data, have fueled renewed interest in EEG research. As graphical summation of electrical potentials of neuronal networks, the EEG provides an immediate measure of mental activity. It has been studied in different mental states and tasks, in stress, and in various psychiatric syndromes. It is especially valuable when precise temporal resolution is required. In cognitive psychology, EEG has advanced researchers' understanding of how the mind works, notably in the areas of attention, memory, and language. Decades after Berger's discovery, modern imaging technologies such as functional magnetic resonance imaging (fMRI) and positron emission tomography (PET) localize biochemical and physical correlates of mental activities with increasing precision. Together with EEG, they explore many of the same conceptual avenues as Berger's early psychophysical work.

Berger's persistence and hard work had overcome many obstacles, but he gained little recognition at home. Amid the political turmoil of Nazi Germany and the outbreak of World War II, his forced retirement, along with a complete ban of any further EEG research, led him to a tragic personal end by suicide.

Bibliography and Suggested Readings

Boutros, Nash, et al., *Standard Electroencephalography in Clinical Psychiatry: A Practical Handbook,* Hoboken: Wiley, 2011.

Borck, Cornelius, "Writing Brains: Tracing the Psyche with the Graphical Method," *History of Psychology* 2005, 8: 79–94.

Borck, Cornelius, "Between Local Cultures and National Styles: Units of Analysis in the History of Electroencephalography," *Comptes Rendus Biologies* May–June 2006, 329(5–6): 450–459.

Gibbs, Frederic A., et al., "The Electroencephalogram in Epilepsy and in Conditions of Impaired Consciousness," *Archives of Neurological Psychiatry* 1935, 34: 1725–1748.

Ginzberg, Raphael, "Three Years with Hans Berger: A Contribution to His Biography," *Journal of the History of Medicine and Allied Sciences* 1949, IV(4): 361–371.

Gloor, Pierre, "Is Berger's Dream Coming True?" *Electroencephalography and Clinical Neurophysiology* 1994, 90(4): 253–266.

Schirmann, Felix, "'The Wondrous Eyes of a New Technology'—A History of the Early Electroencephalography (EEG) of Psychopathy, Delinquency, and Immorality," *Frontiers in Human Neuroscience* 2014, 8: 232.

Electronic Medical Records and Medical Informatics

What	Computerized system of patient medical records and health information.
Where	United States

When	1960s to present
By Whom	Morris Collen (1913–2014); Lawrence Weed (1923–); Donald Lindberg (1933–)
Importance	Provide rapid access to patients' clinical records; to inform and improve therapeutic decisions of healthcare providers and to make available a large pool of anonymous data for research.

The electronic medical record (EMR, or EHR, electronic health record) is transforming 21st-century medical care. A systematic computer-based data repository, the EMR accumulates information concerning the health and care of individual patients. Physicians, nurses, and other healthcare providers record patients' medical history, demographics, medications, test results, physical findings, diagnoses, and more. This information is stored and processed and may be retrieved, displayed, and shared in real time within networks between hospitals, clinics, and private practice settings. The objective is to provide easily accessible patient profiles and other clinical documents across medical information systems.

Case history reports have existed since antiquity. These accounts often included extensive clinical detail and were written and disseminated primarily for didactic purposes. Over time, they evolved to serve multiple purposes. By the early 19th century hospitals were establishing paper files, setting down administrative facts and tabulating patient data to document their charitable mission and justify expenditures. These records also served as clinical teaching cases. Of variable quality, they usually described the "history of the disease, the causes producing it, the remedies employed, and the results of the case." They did not, however, aid in direct patient care; for this, physicians kept their own private notebooks. In 1808 New York Hospital began preserving copies of selected case reports in bound medical and surgical volumes. They were used for research and teaching, and by the late 1800s also became a source of legal information in malpractice and insurance cases.

It was not until the early 1900s that real-time bedside patient chart notes, rather than selected retrospective summaries, became the official hospital records. Generally divided into structured sections for admission, progress, and discharge notes, they charted data such as medical and family history, previous and present illness, physical findings, vital signs, laboratory, and other test results. To ensure documentation of relevant facts, standard recording formats were introduced. Section entries were detailed or scanty and were maintained chronologically in bound volumes. For the same patient, medical and surgical inpatient and outpatient services kept separate records. A single patient's medical record could therefore be widely dispersed and difficult to retrieve.

Mayo Clinic physician Henry Plummer was among the first to address the problem of scattered clinical information. In 1907 he introduced an innovative system in which all individual patient data were combined and organized in a single record. Each patient was assigned a unique clinic number, and charting was structured to adhere to a consistent format. Soon after, New York Presbyterian Hospital further refined the unit medical record, and in 1918 the American College of Surgery instituted a standard requirement for hospitals to record basic clinical data on all patients. This included a summary of care and outcomes, and was to supplement quality control measures.

These reforms led to increasingly voluminous stacks of hospital records shelved in medical record rooms, but they did not necessarily make patient data more readily available, intelligible, or legible. Private care information was even more inaccessible because only a fraction of physician offices kept adequate records.

It was to address the problems inherent in paper records that the idea to develop an electronic medical record first emerged. The advent of digital computers in the 1960s prompted physician Morris Collen, who worked for managed care provider Kaiser Permanente and was an early advocate of computers in healthcare, to develop a computerized database for tracking patients' health. Collen's electronic health record included patient screening and laboratory test results; these were entered by means of punched paper cards into a large mainframe computer, then stored, processed, and aggregated into file-management systems.

Kaiser Permanente's innovative database stimulated research and development of computerized medical information systems around the world. Health maintenance organizations and national health insurance systems in the United States and in Europe promoted the idea of recording patient information electronically. The concept of the "Problem Oriented Medical Record," introduced in the late 1960s by University of Vermont physician Lawrence Weed, lent added support to these efforts. Weed's novel approach generated a record that rationalized clinical assessments and decision making and allowed third parties to verify diagnoses independently. Computerized processing of large amounts of data, especially in hierarchically structured databases and decision trees, was ideally suited to collect this complex medical information and discern significant correlations.

The evolution of structured database management systems in the late 1960s fostered development of the first electronic hospital information systems. Initially, large mainframe computers with random-access disc storage integrated complex patient data into a central database. The advent of minicomputers in the 1970s allowed specialty databases to link directly to central mainframe computers in order to integrate and process information for all clinical and ancillary services in large medical centers. An early hierarchical medical database was the Massachusetts General Hospital Utility Multi-Programming System, or MUMPS. The U.S. Department of Defense and Veterans Administration began using a MUMPS-based medical information system in the 1980s, as did the widely used Epic system 20 years later.

Rapid expansion of increasingly complex systems followed. Storage technology improved and costs diminished. As personal computers became part of popular culture, they also gained greater acceptance as work and professional tools. The invention of NLP, or natural language processing, was an important factor in EMR development. Transmitting patient information required converting words into a language retrievable by a computer, a functional and technical process essential for entry, storage, recovery, and investigation of patient data. NLP was needed to understand unstructured medical, nursing, or operative notes; descriptive histories and physical examinations; or diagnostic interpretations of radiological or laboratory findings. It allowed English (or other language) words, when entered on the computer keyboard or spoken, to be encoded, understood, and categorized.

The advent of the Internet and of World Wide Web communications in the 1990s amplified these advances. Wide-area networks, cloud storage, and supercomputers have made biomedical information accessible to databases worldwide, facilitating multidisciplinary research and discovery of new knowledge.

In the 21st century, development of EMR systems has greatly accelerated. In 2010, U.S. government grants speeded the implementation of computer-based clinical information systems in hospitals and medical offices. By 2012, over half of practicing physicians in the United States reported using electronic medical records instead of traditional handwritten charts.

EMRs stockpile a wealth of individual patient data, function as administrative tools for billing, and serve as a legal record. Clinical observations, physical exams, laboratory results, and digital images are categorized and stored to record patient status, monitor progress, and inform other members of the care team. In a given system, a patient's complete electronic health record may include information derived from multiple clinical sites within a geographic region, thus allowing the sharing of disparate clinical data and, in theory, improving communication and coordination of care.

Ideally, electronic medical records will aid in medical decision making, help improve patient care, and assist in patient–provider interaction. However, actual performance of many commercial EMR systems has fallen short of expectations. Practitioners complain they are not user friendly, that reporting and data analysis tools are cumbersome, and that many systems lag behind other technological innovations. In addition, costs can be prohibitive, especially for solo practitioners, forcing them into group practice. Data entry presents another hurdle for providers not proficient in keyboard typing. Voice recognition software can circumvent this, but at a cost. Some practices have resorted to resuscitating professional "scribes," an expedient that introduces another person into a confidential physician–patient relationship and may significantly alter communication.

The introduction of electronic medical records has had an enormous impact on modern medical practice. Technological challenges are ongoing, and the full benefits of EMRs have yet to be assessed.

Bibliography and Suggested Readings

Collen, Morris, *Computer Medical Databases: The First Six Decades (1950–2010)*, London: Springer, 2012.

Collen, Morris, and Ball, Marion, eds., *The History of Medical Informatics in the United States*, 2nd ed., London: Springer, 2015.

Gillum, Richard, "From Papyrus to the Electronic Tablet: A Brief History of the Clinical Medical Record with Lessons for the Digital Age," *The American Journal of Medicine* October 2013, 126(10): 853–857.

Siegler, Eugenia, "The Evolving Medical Record," *Annals of Internal Medicine* 2010, 153: 671–677.

Magnetic Resonance Imaging (MRI)

What	An advanced medical imaging technique using strong electromagnetic fields to manipulate the components of specific atomic nuclei. Computer analysis of the energy emitted during this process provides spatial information used to derive images of structures that cannot otherwise be visualized.
Where	United States; United Kingdom
When	1970s
By Whom	Raymond Damadian (b. 1936); Paul Lauterbur (1929–2007); Sir Peter Mansfield (b.1933)
Importance	Made possible detailed images of internal anatomical structures, soft tissue injuries, or diseases; generally considered preferable to computed tomography (CT) because it does not expose the body to ionizing radiation and has no known adverse effects.

In medicine, imaging of internal organs with noninvasive methods has become increasingly important for both diagnosis and treatment. Magnetic resonance imaging, or MRI, was a major breakthrough for late-20th-century medical research and diagnostics. MRI exploits the response, or *resonance*, of the hydrogen atom to electromagnetic energy. Hydrogen atoms are the usual source of resonance, because hydrogen (as a part of water molecules) is the most prevalent element in the human body.

The proton located in the nucleus of the hydrogen atom has fundamental magnetic properties. When strong electromagnetic energy is applied at the appropriate resonant frequency, the excited proton absorbs the energy and changes its steady-state orientation. When the magnetic induction changes or stops, the proton relaxes and returns to its original state. In the course of this process it emits a radio frequency signal registered by a receiver. These transmitted electromagnetic signals are used to construct internal images of the body by computerized axial tomography. Contrast between different tissues is determined by the rate at which the excited atoms return to their state of equilibrium.[1]

The idea that atomic particles could be manipulated in such a way originated with the work of Austrian physicist Wolfgang Pauli in 1924. In 1937, Columbia professor Isidor Rabi recognized that atomic nuclei respond to a strong magnetic field and rotate with a frequency dependent on the strength of this field. Rabi coined the phrase *nuclear magnetic resonance*, or NMR, for this magnetic movement, or spin, of the atomic nucleus.

The resonance phenomenon is governed by a simple relationship between magnetic energy and radio wave frequency. For every atomic nucleus, there is a mathematical constant, which determines wavelength as a function of the strength of the magnetic field. Two American scientists, Felix Bloch at Stanford and Edward Purcell at Harvard, demonstrated this phenomenon in 1946. They independently made the first successful nuclear magnetic resonance experiments in which they found that nucleic protons resonate to magnetic induction at the specific radio frequency of the particular atom. Because the resonance frequency is specific to each substance, NMR can determine its chemical composition and structure.

---

1. Two signals are recorded: the relaxation times T1 and T2, which measure the net intervals for the components of the excited nuclei to return to equilibrium. T1 measures the relaxation time for the component parallel to the external field, and T2 that for the component perpendicular to this field. The relative difference between T1 and T2 at various points corresponds to differences in adjacent tissues, from which inferred images are then constructed.

Bloch and Purcell were awarded the Nobel Prize for Physics in 1952 for their discovery. Their work led to NMR spectroscopy, which became widely used to study the microscopic structure of molecules and the composition of chemical compounds using small magnets.

In the late 1960s, State University of New York (SUNY) physician Raymond Damadian began investigating the use of NMR in the detection of cancer. His work, although controversial, was instrumental in the introduction of NMR into medical imaging and research. Damadian departed from observations that tumor cells differed from normal cells because they contain more water and thus more hydrogen atoms. He tested his theory on rats with cancer and demonstrated that NMR signals of cancerous tissue samples differed from those of healthy tissues. He published his results in 1971 and subsequently developed a full-body scanning device, which he named the *Indomitable*, claiming it to be a machine capable of detecting cancer.

At the same time Paul Lauterbur, professor of chemistry at SUNY at Stony Brook, discovered that variations in magnetic fields could be used to determine the location of protons in space. Working on NMR imaging of water molecules, he found that hydrogen atoms placed in a strong magnetic field align themselves like the needles of a compass. When they return to their original position, they emit radio waves that can be analyzed to determine their origin. Lauterbur's key insight was that spatial information could be gathered by applying magnetic field gradients in all three dimensions. These data could then be used to create two- or three-dimensional MRI images of molecular structures that could not otherwise be visualized. In 1973 Lauterbur described the new technique—he called it "zeugmatography" (from the Greek meaning joining together)—in a seminal paper published in *Nature*. His idea revolutionized NMR imaging.

British scientist Peter Mansfield, who later shared the 2003 Nobel Prize in Physiology or Medicine with Lauterbur, further expanded the utilization of gradients in the magnetic field. He showed that MRI signals could be mathematically analyzed, which helped to refine their interpretation and made possible the creation of detailed images. He also developed a technique called echo-planar imaging, which allowed for much faster collection of images. This greatly increased MRI use in clinical applications. In neuroimaging it led to functional MRI (fMRI), which measures neuronal stimulation and cerebral activity by detecting associated changes in cerebral blood flow.

In the 21st century magnetic resonance imaging has become routine in the evaluation of many disease processes, often replacing CT. Both are tomographic techniques allowing noninvasive diagnosis. However, CT images only reflect the physical density of tissues traversed by the X-ray beams, whereas MRI differentiates them by their chemical composition. Moreover, MRI does not use ionizing radiation, which can damage DNA and increase cancer risk. Instead, it uses magnetic fields and radio waves, neither of which is known to cause cell damage. MRI further produces high-resolution images, distinguishing tissues in any imaging plane. It provides not only detailed anatomical and morphological data, but can collect functional data such as variations in cerebral blood flow as different tasks are performed.

MRI has become the method of choice in neuroimaging. It allows visualization of small tumors and differentiates between gray and white matter, facilitating diagnosis of many central nervous system diseases. Further applications include real-time MR fluoroscopy and open MRI, which make possible *in vivo* interventions.

Generally safe, MRI is contraindicated in patients harboring any metallic foreign bodies such as surgical implants or shrapnel.

Bibliography and Suggested Readings

Gunderman, Richard B., *X-Ray Vision: The Evolution of Medical Imaging and Its Human Significance*, Oxford: Oxford University Press, 2013.

Kevles, Bettyann H., *Naked to the Bone: Medical Imaging in the Twentieth Century*, New Brunswick: Rutgers University Press, 1997.

Magnetic Resonance, www.magnetic-resonance.org.

Rinck, Peter A., *Magnetic Resonance in Medicine. The Basic Textbook of the European Magnetic Resonance Forum,* 7th ed., 2013. Electronic version 7.1; October 1, 2013. Original publication Oxford, Boston: Blackwell Scientific Publications, 1993.

Pap Smear

What	Screening test performed to detect cancer or precancerous lesions on the surface of the uterine cervix.
Where	United States
When	1928; 1941
By Whom	George Papanicolaou (1883–1962)
Importance	One of the most significant 20th-century advances in early cervical cancer detection; highlighted the importance of exfoliative cytology in pathological science.

The Papanicolaou, or Pap, smear, also known as cervicovaginal cytology, has been the major screening tool for cervical cancer for over half a century. The test is simple, inexpensive, and minimally invasive. During the procedure, a speculum is inserted into the vaginal canal to open it and visualize the cervix. The outer surface of the cervix is then scraped with a small spatula to collect a cell sample from the transformation zone, where the squamous cell lining meets the inner glandular cells and where precancerous changes are known to occur. Recent devices such as the endocervical brush improve sampling of cells from the cervical opening.

The collected cells are inspected for abnormal features indicative of precancerous change. Precursor lesions of cervical cancer often appear considerably earlier than manifest localized or invasive carcinoma. Therefore, the recognition of abnormal dysplastic or neoplastic cells and prompt intervention can prevent full-blown disease.

Initially, specimens were smeared onto glass microscopic slides and then fixed and stained with the Papanicolaou stain; this produced various cytoplasmic colors depending on cell type and maturity. Now, cell scrapings or brushings are suspended in liquid and sent to a laboratory for slide preparation and examination. This liquid-based technology also allows for further testing, including that for human papillomavirus (HPV) DNA, because only a portion of the sample is used to prepare the slide.

The technique was named for Greek American scientist George Papanicolaou who developed it during his studies of female reproduction. In 1915, shortly after immigrating to the United States, Dr. Papanicolaou, a European-trained physician and zoologist and an expert microscopist, had started to investigate the menstrual cycle of guinea pigs, a species that does not visibly shed tissue during menses. To estimate the proper time for egg retrieval he conceived of using a small nasal speculum placed in their vaginas in order to discern cyclical bleeding. When he examined the animals' exfoliated cervical cells, he found recurring changes that corresponded precisely to their ovarian hormonal cycles.

In 1920, Dr. Papanicolaou began studying cytological patterns and their correlation to hormonal changes in women. His own wife Andromache was to be his first, and long-term, experimental subject, and Papanicolaou reportedly tested her vaginal smears daily. He also collected cell scrapings of gynecological patients at Cornell University Clinic. In 1925, with funds from the National Research Council and the Maternal Health Committee, he recruited 12 hospital staff volunteers, together with a number of pregnant gynecological and surgical patients, for a systematic study of cervical cell morphology. Participants were tested regularly to determine normal hormonal changes and to diagnose early pregnancy.

It was the unexpected finding of malignant cells in one of his samples— Papanicolaou later recollected this as "one of the most thrilling experiences" in his career—which led him to explore the value of this method in cancer detection. He began to gather additional data from women with various pathological conditions and found that in cervical cancer, many abnormal cells were shed and could be readily identified by cytological study of patients' vaginal smears.

Papanicolaou presented the results of his investigations at the 1928 "Third Race Betterment Conference" in Battle Creek, Michigan, but there was little interest in his new method of cancer diagnosis. Cervical biopsies, it was argued, were far more precise than crude smears. In France during the same year, Roumanian pathologist Aurel Babes had published his study of a small sample of extracted cervical specimens. However, his method, described as an alternative to tissue sectioning for pathological diagnosis of localized carcinoma, differed both in sampling and processing.

The medical profession by and large ignored these discoveries. The Pap test was not put to clinical use until more than 10 years later when Papanicolaou, together with gynecological pathologist Herbert Traut, and with the support of the new chair of the Cornell Anatomy Department, started a clinical trial in which routine vaginal smears were performed on all new gynecological admissions to New York Hospital. Cytological examination of these samples uncovered a number of previously unsuspected, asymptomatic uterine cancers. Some were at such an early, superficial stage that they could not be otherwise diagnosed.

In 1941 and 1943, Papanicolaou and Traut published the results of their studies in a landmark report, followed by a descriptive atlas of normal and pathological cells in vaginal smears. They emphasized the need for a simple diagnostic tool to detect early cancer and precancerous epithelial changes and described the details of their method. Their work was to change the practice of gynecology. Over the ensuing decade, the American Cancer Society started a program to educate professionals about the preventive value of the Pap smear. Papanicolaou began teaching cytology at Cornell Medical College, and other training programs in cytopathology followed. By 1950, both the National Cancer Institute and the American Cancer Society had initiated mass screening campaigns. Their results made plain the value of the new test in detecting early cervical lesions. Before, exfoliated cervicovaginal cells had been discarded, but now their importance in diagnosis and prevention was established. Papanicolaou, with his disciples, eventually extended the original technique for specimen collection and staining to other body sites.

Today, cytology screening has become computer assisted. Cells are analyzed with morphological interpretation software. Slides with high numbers of abnormal cells are ranked and manually reviewed by cytotechnologists. Criteria for classifying results have been refined. Yet, the method is far from perfect and has been criticized for only moderate sensitivity, with false-negative rates as high as 25 percent due to either sampling errors or failure to identify abnormal cells.

To address these concerns, supplementary tests, mainly for human papillomavirus DNA, have been added to cytology-based screening alone. In the United States, the American College of Obstetricians and Gynecologists, the Preventive Services Task Force, and the American Cancer Society now recommend routine screening for cervical cancer with Pap smear every three years for women 21 to 65, or HPV testing together with Pap smear for women 30 to 65 every five years.

George Papanicolaou was internationally recognized for his accomplishments; between 1948 and 1953 he was nominated 18 times for the Nobel Prize. When his test was first introduced, cervical cancer was the number one killer of women worldwide. Since then, Pap screening has greatly reduced cervical cancer mortality. Still, the disease remains one of the world's deadliest preventable cancers. It is responsible for an estimated 270,000 deaths annually, most of which occur in developing countries.

Bibliography and Suggested Readings

Diamantis, Aristidis, et al., "What's in a Name? Evidence That Papanicolaou, Not Babes, Deserves Credit for the Pap Test," *Diagnostic Cytopathology* 2010, 38: 473–476.

Koss, Leopold, "Letters to the Editor: Aurel Babes," *International Journal of Gynecological Pathology* January 2003, 22(1): 101–102.

Mukherjee, Siddhartha, *The Emperor of All Maladies: A Biography of Cancer*, New York: Scribner, 2010.

Papanicolaou, George, "New Cancer Diagnosis," *Proceedings of the Third Race Betterment Conference*, Battle Creek, Michigan, 1928: 528.

Shepard, Elizabeth M., 2011, "George Papanicolaou: Development of the Pap Smear," http://weill.cornell.edu/archives/blog/2011/06/george-papanicolaou-development -of-the-pap-smear.html.

Tambouret, Rosemary, "The Evolution of the Papanicolaou Smear," *Clinical Obstetrics and Gynecology* March 2013, 56(1): 3–9.

U.S. Preventive Services Task Force, 2012, "Final Recommendation Statement," http:// www.uspreventiveservicestaskforce.org/Page/Document/RecommendationState mentFinal/cervical-cancer-screening#consider.

Vilos, George, "The History of the Papanicolaou Smear and the Odyssey of George and Andromache Papanicolaou," *Obstetrics and Gynecology* March 1998, 91(3): 479–483.

Sphygmomanometer

What	Instrument designed to measure blood pressure.
Where	England; Italy; Russia
When	1733; 1896; 1905
By Whom	Stephen Hales (1677–1761); Scipione Riva-Rocci (1863–1937); Nikolai Korotkoff (1874–1920)
Importance	Important technological innovation allowing the study of physiological blood pressure ranges; improved assessment of cardiovascular function.

Study of the pulse and its pressure was long considered an art and called for qualitative assessments to be made only by experts. In the modern era, quantitative measuring of blood pressure became part of wide-ranging attempts to apply scientific methods to the study of the body and how it functioned. The sphygmomanometer was one of the devices developed to record blood pressure, a normal, vital function.

Blood pressure is the force exerted by the circulating blood upon the walls of the arteries. This pressure originates in the pumping action of the heart, and its waves can be felt wherever arterial vessels lie near the body surface, such as the wrist, neck, elbow crease, or groin. Large arteries always have a certain constant internal pressure because blood courses through them more quickly than through small vessels and capillary beds can absorb it. Contraction of the heart muscle, or *systole*, causes the blood pressure to rise to its highest point; relaxation, or *diastole*, brings the pressure down to its lowest point. Usually, the pressure in the brachial (arm) artery serves as a standard. It is conventionally measured in millimeters of mercury. Multiple factors can influence blood pressure levels, and normal readings vary with physical activity, emotional stress, and age. The average for healthy young people is generally considered to be 120 mm Hg for systolic and 80 mm Hg for diastolic pressure.

The first measuring of blood pressure dates back to the 1730s when English clergyman and scientist Stephen Hales inserted a narrow brass pipe into the femoral artery of a horse. Affixing to this a long glass tube of similar diameter and then untying the ligature of the artery, he was able to observe the "force of the blood," which rose up in the tube by nearly nine feet above the level of the left ventricle, as well as its rise and fall with each pulse beat. Hales described his experiment in a 1733 volume entitled *Haemostaticks* but eventually abandoned further blood pressure investigations on account of the "disagreeableness of Anatomical dissections."

It took another century for detailed blood pressure study to resume. In 1828 French physician and physicist Jean Poiseuille, best known for his work on the viscosity of fluids, introduced a mercury manometer (instrument using a column of liquid to measure pressure) for the measurement of arterial blood pressure. When connecting his manometer to a small cannula filled with an anticoagulant and inserted directly into an artery, he was able to demonstrate that pressure was maintained in arteries as small as 2 mm. The 1847 kymograph of German physiologist Carl Ludwig was inspired by Poiseuille's device. Ludwig used the same manometer and cannula system, but added a floating stylus, which could inscribe pressure waves onto a revolving cylinder, thus in effect founding the graphical method of recording clinical data.

All these instruments, however, required arterial puncture in order to determine pressures. In 1855, German physician Karl von Vierordt proposed the first indirect, noninvasive technique to determine arterial pressure. His apparatus, later refined by French scientist Etienne Jules Marey, measured the external counter pressure necessary to obliterate blood flow and cause pulsations to cease by means of a weight attached to the lever of a sphygmograph.

It was Austrian physician Karl Ritter von Basch (1837–1905) who developed the first aneroid sphygmomanometer using an inflatable rubber bag filled with water and connected to a mercury-filled manometer bulb. The bag was applied over the pulse until distal pulsations stopped, at which point the systolic pressure was recorded by measuring the rise of the column of mercury. This instrument was much more accurate than previous devices. It also demonstrated hemodynamic changes in certain pathological conditions, such as lowered blood pressure in patients with fever and markedly elevated pressures in patients with obstructive arteriosclerosis. Basch was one of the first to compile systematic clinical data using his machine. Study of the pulse thus became linked to blood pressure monitoring.

In 1896, Italian physician Scipione Riva-Rocci introduced what is considered the prototype of modern-day sphygmomanometry. Riva-Rocci had studied the work of Vierordt, Marey, and Basch, and from 1896 to 1897 published a series of articles on his new method for measuring blood pressure. Previous practice entailed compression of the radial pulse, whereas Riva-Rocci's innovation consisted of compressing the brachial artery just above the elbow. An inflatable rubber band was wrapped around the arm and pumped up until the pulse disappeared, after which air was released until the pulse reappeared; both readings were noted. Disappearance of the pulse on palpation corresponded to the systolic arterial pressure, as Riva-Rocci confirmed by calibration experiments in animals and with human cadavers.

The new instrument enabled easy measurement of (systolic) blood pressure in clinical practice and was gradually introduced and adopted worldwide. In 1901 noted Johns Hopkins neurosurgeon Harvey Cushing became acquainted with Riva-Rocci's device and contributed to its introduction in American medical practice. Subsequent data on the important role of circulatory pressures in shock prompted Cushing to institute blood pressure monitoring during his surgical operations; according to some observers, this gradually led to a general acceptance of blood pressure measuring in clinical medicine.

In 1905, soon after the introduction of Riva-Rocci's technique, Russian surgeon Nikolai Korotkoff began using a stethoscope applied to the brachial artery below the cuff in order to monitor pulse pressure sounds. He discovered that a fully constricted artery did not emit any sounds, but that as pressure in the inflated cuff declined and the mercury in the manometer dropped to a certain height, there appeared faint pulse tones indicating that a portion of the bloodstream had passed under the sleeve. The point at which the first sound appeared thus corresponded to the maximum (systolic) pressure. Finally, with further release of pressure and fall of the column of mercury, all pulse sounds disappeared; this reflected free flow and occurred at a point when the minimum arterial pressure was greater than the pressure in the sleeve. This point was coincident with cardiac expansion, or diastole. Korotkoff's auscultatory method thus allowed simple and accurate determination of both systolic and diastolic arterial pressure.

Today, the noninvasive measuring of blood pressure has become part of the standard patient examination and is accepted as an important vital sign in the diagnostic assessment. Present-day sphygmomanometers range from mercurial to aneroid or digital models, and technical advances have improved accuracy and ease of use. In hospital settings, blood pressure can be measured continuously by local sensors and sophisticated electronic pressure gauges. Its monitoring is an essential part of routine perioperative care of all patients.

Few discoveries have had such a significant impact on everyday clinical medical practice. In the 21st century, hypertension, a condition in which blood pressure is persistently higher than the norm, affects millions of people throughout the world. Most cases are those of so-called "essential hypertension," where the cause is unknown. Yet, blood pressure is one of the most important predictors of life expectancy. Treatment of hypertension reduces the incidence of stroke, heart attack, and kidney disease. Accurate measurement and regular monitoring of blood pressure are therefore essential.

Bibliography and Suggested Readings

Booth, Jeremy, "A Short History of Blood Pressure Measurement," *Proceedings of the Royal Society of Medicine* 1977, 70(11): 793–799.

Lederer, Susan E., *Flesh and Blood: Organ Transplantation and Blood Transfusion in 20th Century America*, Oxford: Oxford University Press, 2008.

Murphy, Fred T., "Report on Blood-Pressure Observations at the Massachusetts General Hospital," *Boston Medical and Surgical Journal* 1904, 150: 264–269.

Naqvi, Nassim H., and Blaufox, M. Donald, *Blood Pressure Measurement: An Illustrated History*, New York: Parthenon, 1998.

Noyes, Bradford, "The History of the Thermometer and the Sphygmomanometer," *Bulletin of the Medical Library Association* 1936, 24(3): 155–165.

Stethoscope

What	Acoustic device for listening to the internal sounds of the human body; mostly used to listen to heart and lung sounds and to arterial blood flow.
Where	Paris, France
When	1816
By Whom	René T. H. Laënnec (1781–1826)
Importance	Significant advance in diagnostic practice; major influence on the emerging science of pathological anatomy and on concepts of disease.

A key contribution to 19th-century clinical medicine was that of French physician René Théophile Hyacinthe Laënnec, the inventor of the stethoscope. Laënnec, who had studied medicine under several prominent teachers, including Dupuytren and Corvisart, both personal physicians to Napoleon, was working at the Necker Hospital in Paris when he introduced his new device. In his now famous *Treatise on Mediate Auscultation* he described his discovery:

> I was consulted in 1816 for a young woman who presented with symptoms of a diseased heart, and in whom palpation and percussion yielded few results because of her plumpness. Since the age and gender of the patient did not permit the type of examination I have just mentioned (direct application of the ear to the chest), I came to recall a well known acoustic phenomenon: if one places the ear against one end of a wooden log, one can hear very distinctly the tap of a pin at the other

end. It occurred to me that one might perhaps make use of this physical property in the case at hand. I took a paper notebook, shaped it into a tightly compressed roll, one end of which I applied to the precordial region, and, putting my ear to the other end, I was as surprised as I was gratified to hear the beating of the heart with much greater clarity and distinctness than I had ever been able to before by the direct application of the ear.

He called his discovery "mediate auscultation"—indirect listening, or listening by means of a medium, or instrument, to sounds produced inside the body—as contrasted to "immediate auscultation," then the usual method of placing one's ear onto the patient's chest wall.

Laënnec quickly understood that this method could become a useful tool, "to be applied not only to the study of the heart beats, but to that of all the movements that can produce sound within the chest cavity, and consequently to the exploration of respiration, of the voice, the râle (a sibilant, rattling sound heart in auscultation of the chest), and perhaps even of the fluctuations of liquid spread within the pleura or the pericardium."

Initially Laënnec called his instrument simply "*le cylindre*" (the cylinder), not imagining it would be necessary to give a name to such a plain, artless device. The term "stethoscope" (from the Greek *stethos*, chest, and *skopein*, to explore or to examine) first appeared in the thesis of one of his students in 1818. The early stethoscopes were indeed cylinders, about one foot in length and over an inch thick, made of tightly rolled notebooks and wrapped in gummed paper. Later Laënnec devised a cylinder made of wood with a central canal and a funnel-shaped hollow end. About nine inches long, it had two parts that could be unscrewed for easier carrying.

Laënnec's clinical position at the Hôpital Necker allowed him to compare sounds heard with his new instrument with *post mortem* findings at autopsy. Departing from these observations he painstakingly constructed signs that would be specific and sensitive for given diagnostic entities. Many of the terms he coined to describe particular auscultatory phenomena—such as *pectoriloquy*, *egophony*, *rhonchi*, and *râles*—are still used in medicine today to characterize physical findings.

Laënnec's stethoscope revolutionized diagnostic examination of the chest. The carefully elaborated new knowledge of the nature of heart, breath, and chest sounds in different pathological conditions laid the foundation for modern diagnosis of chest diseases. Illnesses that until then had only been known by the patient's symptoms—fever, cough, pain, difficulty breathing, or hemoptysis, the spitting of blood—could now be described by their relationship to underlying anatomical structures: bronchitis, pneumonia, pleuritis, and many others, including the many signs of pulmonary tuberculosis, a major scourge of the era. Physicians' ability to correlate pathological changes in the chest with their own auscultatory findings was a breakthrough, which established the stethoscope as a powerful noninvasive diagnostic tool.

The stethoscope became a valuable adjunct in teaching clinical diagnosis, and the many foreign students drawn to the Paris clinics were quick to spread word of the new technique. Importantly, Laënnec's approach demonstrated the importance of scientific investigation in the diagnostic process. Observations alone did not constitute theory. Medical science was not simple accumulation of facts, but required a system to link the information gathered and a method to understand and develop underlying principles. One of the major medical innovations of the 19th century, Laënnec's stethoscope thus became an early symbol of the scientific medical profession.

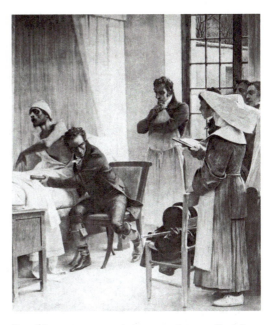

René Laënnec examining a patient at Paris' Necker Hospital, 1816. Laënnec's stethoscope greatly improved both the acoustics and ease of auscultation. It also helped the physician maintain a polite distance from patients of different gender or class, or from bodies that were "unclean or bathed in sweat" where direct application of the ear to the chest would "naturally inspire repugnance," preventing the examiner's "habitual and frequent use of this method of exploration." (Bettmann/ Getty Images)

But not all physicians were ready to embrace the new method. In the United States, where the *New England Journal of Medicine* had reported Laënnec's invention as early as 1821, acceptance was slow. L. A. Conner, a founder of the American Heart Association and a meticulous clinician, is said to have practiced immediate auscultation as late as 1932; he examined his patients with his ear placed on a "sounding towel" draped over their chest.

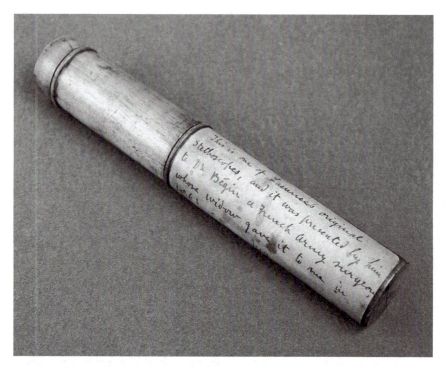

Photograph of one of René Laënnec's original stethoscopes, ca. 1820. Made of wood and brass, it consists of a single hollow tube. The familiar binaural stethoscope, with rubber tubing going to both ears, was not developed until the 1850s. Laënnec demonstrated the importance of the instrument in diagnosing diseases of the heart and lungs, and his stethoscope came to symbolize a new clinical approach to medicine at the turn of the nineteenth century. (Science & Society Picture Library/Getty Images)

Laënnec's stethoscope was a single monaural tube. In 1851, Irish physician Arthur Leared invented a binaural stethoscope, and in 1852 American George Cammann perfected this design for commercial production. A version developed by Rappaport and Sprague in the 1940s consisted of two sides, one of which is used for the respiratory system, the other for the cardiovascular system. It became the standard until the early 1960s when David Littmann, a Harvard cardiologist, created a lighter stethoscope with better acoustics.

Tuberculosis had been the primary focus of Laënnec's clinical studies and was the disease that ultimately killed him; he died at the premature age of 45. There was no autopsy, but his cousin who had examined him with his stethoscope during his final weeks, reported finding auscultatory evidence of pulmonary cavities.

Bibliography and Suggested Readings

Duffin, Jacalyn, *To See with a Better Eye: A Life of R.T.H. Laennec*, Princeton: Princeton University Press, 1998.

Roguin, Ariel, "René Théophile Hyacinthe Laënnec (1781–1826): The Man Behind the Stethoscope," *Clinical Medicine & Research* 2006, 4(3): 230–235.

Théophile Hyacinthe Laënnec, René, *De l'auscultation médiate, ou, Traité du diagnostic des maladies des poumons et du coeur: fondé principalement sur ce nouveau moyen d'exploration*, Paris: J.-A. Brosson, et J.-S. Chaudé, 1819: 7–8.

Thermometer

What	An instrument used to measure body temperature; traditionally inserted under the patient's tongue, armpit, or into the anus, it gives readings of oral, axillary, or rectal temperatures.
Where	Italy; Holland; England
When	1612; 1717; 1867
By Whom	Santorio Santorii (1561–1636); Daniel Gabriel Fahrenheit (1686–1736); Carl August Wunderlich (1815–1877); Thomas Clifford Allbutt (1836–1925)
Importance	Valuable tool in clinical diagnosis providing an objective measure of normal or abnormal body temperature, especially of fever, the hallmark of many infectious and other disease conditions.

Among symptoms of disease, changes in body temperature have always been known to be an essential part of clinical observation. In ancient times, fever and its patterns of rise and fall, such as the tertian or quartan (every third or fourth day) paroxysms of malarial fever, were recognized to be important markers. Fever was considered not just a cardinal sign of acute illness, but a disease entity in itself. It was explained by the doctrine of the four humors, and ways to alleviate it were part and parcel of Hippocratic practice.

Before the advent of the thermometer, the physician used the touch of his hand to determine the body's warmth. In 1612, Sanctorius, professor of medicine at Padua, also known as Santorio Santorii, perfected Galileo's rudimentary early water thermoscope by adding a numerical scale in order to measure the difference between normal and abnormal body temperature. He was the first to introduce a mouth thermometer for the use in disease. Scientific measurement was achieved in the late 17th century when the Dutch natural philosopher and polymath Christiaan Huygens developed the parameters of the centigrade system, basing them on the freezing and boiling points of water. In 1717, Daniel Gabriel Fahrenheit devised a scale with smaller increments of 180 degrees between these reference points. He used mercury rather than water because of its more rapid expansion and contraction.

Dutch physician Hermann Boerhaave and his students Gerhard van Swieten and Anton de Haen pioneered the regular use of thermometry in clinical practice. Their observations on the diurnal changes of temperature in healthy individuals, the relationship of temperature to pulse rate, and the effect of shivering (which produces a rise in temperature) led them to monitor temperature changes during the course of illness. They soon recommended that fever be measured with a thermometer rather than estimated by manual touch. Van Swieten, by then professor of medicine at the University of Vienna, used Fahrenheit's mercurial thermometer and applied it to both mouth and axilla.

The early years of clinical thermometry were hampered by the lack of accurate instruments. In addition, although the number of clinical investigations was increasing, there were as yet no general principles derived from those studies that would justify the use of the thermometer in everyday practice. But by the mid-19th century scientific study on the chemistry and physics of body heat production and regulation was underway. Antoine Lavoisier, Hermann von Helmholtz, James Joule, Claude Bernard, and Gustave Hirn were among the many researchers who contributed to the understanding of thermal changes in both physiological and pathological processes. In medicine, it was largely through the work of Carl August Wunderlich, professor at the University of Leipzig, that physicians came to understand that fever was not a disease, but only a sign of disease, and that measuring the patient's temperature was as important as recording his pulse.

Wunderlich was the first to establish normal temperature ranges (36.2 to 37.5 on the Celsius scale) after studying temperature fluctuations in thousands of clinical cases. He noted variations both in physiological states—diurnal changes in the healthy individual; variations in menstruation, pregnancy, and childbirth—as well as in acute diseases such as typhus, smallpox, measles, scarlet fever, tonsillitis, meningitis, and pneumonia. He published his findings in 1868 and concluded that "a physician who practiced without employing a thermometer was like a blind man trying to distinguish colors by feeling." Wunderlich demonstrated that body temperature remained fairly constant in

On the Development of the Thermometer and Its Uses

... For the past sixteen years my attention has been uninterruptedly directed to the course pursued by the temperature in diseases of various kinds. The thermometer has been regularly employed at least twice daily, and in febrile patients from four to eight times a days, and even oftener, ... for all the patients in my wards .... In this way I have gradually gathered a material, which comprises many thousand cases of thermometric observations of disease .... The more my observations were multiplied, the more firmly rooted did my conviction become of the unparalleled value of this method of investigation, as giving an accurate and reliable insight into the condition of the sick ...

... My immediate purpose has been to write a practical book, and to lay before my medical brethren ... the eminent usefulness of thermometric observations. A knowledge of the course of temperature in disease is highly important to the medical practitioner, and, indeed, indispensable:

Because all the phenomena of the sick are deserving of study

Because the temperature can be determined with an ease which is common to few other phenomena

Because the temperature can neither be feigned nor falsified

Because we may conclude the presence of some disturbance in the [body's] economy from the mere fact of altered temperatures; ...

Because the height of the temperature often decides both the degree and the danger of the attack

Because thermometric observation may serve to aid in the discovery of the laws regulating the course of certain diseases, and may enable us to learn them

Because when once the normal course of certain diseases has been determined, thermometry is able to simplify, confirm, and certify the diagnosis

Because thermometric investigations indicate most rapidly and most safely any deviations from the regular course of the disease

Because the behavior of the temperature during the progress of the disease discovers to us both relapses and ameliorations before we should otherwise recognize them

Because in this way thermometry is able to relate the results of our therapeutic efforts

Because it puts us on our guard against the injurious influences which affect our patients in the course of their illness

Because it is able to indicate the transition from one stage of the disease into another, and particularly the commencement of convalescence and its complete establishment

Because it reveals the existence of complications, and shows how far recovery is from being yet complete

Because it generally reveals the fact of a fatal termination being imminent

Because it often announces . . . a fatal prognosis with great distinctness

And lastly, because it furnishes a certain proof of the reality of death, when this is otherwise uncertain.

If I succeed in diffusing . . . the conviction of the truth of these propositions . . . the object of my work is already obtained.

Dr. Wunderlich
Leipzic; March, 1868.

Source: Wunderlich, Carl A., *On the Temperature in Diseases: A Manual of Medical Thermometry*, translated from the second German edition. London: New Sydenham Society, 1871.

health but that there was great variation in disease. Moreover, he showed that the course of certain diseases correlated to specific temperature variations. His carefully compiled statistics (he estimated having taken several million thermometric readings in about 25,000 patients!) established the definitive importance of accurate thermometry in clinical diagnosis, prognosis, and treatment regimen.

Wunderlich's systematic temperature recordings had been obtained by means of large, bulky thermometers, which required a long time to register accurately. Recognizing the need for a more practical instrument, English physician Thomas Clifford Allbutt in 1867 invented a clinical thermometer approximately six inches in length that physicians could easily carry in a pocket. Previous mercury-in-glass devices had been a foot long and cumbersome to use (patients had to be in contact with the device for about 20 minutes), but Allbutt's version was convenient and portable and provided accurate readings within five minutes. Made freely available by its inventor, it was rapidly disseminated and widely adopted.

By the end of the 19th century, with the encouragement of the medical establishment, use of the clinical thermometer had spread from the hospital to family practitioners and nurses and to the home. The American physician Edward Séguin in his 1873 *Manual of Thermometry, for Mothers, Nurses, and All Who Have Charge of the Young and of the Sick* wrote that the appreciation of the temperature of the body took precedence "over everything else in the art of taking care of children and patients generally." He advocated educating women in the "handling, recording and intelligent reading" of the medical thermometer and encouraged his colleagues to "make them love, study and trust the little instrument which—like the little finger of the fairy tale—tells things that no one can know otherwise . . ."

Wunderlich's findings had enabled physicians to link extremes of temperature with specific illnesses. The new portable thermometer, which allowed simple and routine recording and charting of patients' temperatures, provided important objective data documenting the course of an illness. Fever curves were not only visual guides to diagnosis and treatment, but also important prognostic indicators. Together with the stethoscope, the original Allbutt Clinical Thermometer became an indispensable diagnostic aid in the doctor's armamentarium.

Allbutt's basic thermometer is still in use today, although recent advances in design have included digital, electronic, and infrared thermometers. In 1964 Theodore Benzinger developed the ear thermometer, and in 1984 David Phillips invented the infrared ear thermometer.

Today, research has shown that fever is not just a sign of disease but also an important mechanism in the body's natural defense against infection. The febrile response is thought to assist the healing process by increasing mobility and stimulating phagocytic action of white blood cells and by diminishing the effects of bacterial toxins. Its recognition and study, made possible by the advent of the medical thermometer, are therefore all the more important.

Bibliography and Suggested Readings

Haller, John S., "Medical Thermometry—A Short History," *Western Journal of Medicine* January 1985, 142: 108–116.

Hippocrates, *On Regimen in Acute Diseases*, Appendix Part 1, http://classics.mit.edu//Hippocrates/acutedis.html.

Wunderlich, Carl A., *On the Temperature in Diseases: A Manual of Medical Thermometry*, translated from the second German edition by W. Bathurst Woodman, London: The New Sydenham Society, 1871.

Ultrasound

What	Medical ultrasound is a diagnostic imaging technique using ultrasound waves to visualize internal organs and other body structures to define normal anatomy or detect possible pathology.
Where	Italy; France; Austria; England; United States; Sweden
When	1877; 1940s and 1950s
By Whom	Pierre Curie (1859–1906); Paul Langevin (1872–1946); Douglas Howry (1920–1969); John J. Wild (1914–2009); Ian Donald (1910–1987); Inge Edler (1911–2001); Hellmuth Hertz (1920–1990)
Importance	Widely used aid in medical diagnosis; obstetric ultrasound is an important tool to monitor fetal development or pregnancy complications.

Ultrasonography, the making of images by ultrasound, is an imaging technology that relies on sound waves to create two- and three-dimensional images in order to visualize internal structures in the human body. In physics, the term applies to high-frequency nonaudible sound waves above 20 kHz. The normal range of human hearing is approximately 20 to 20,000 Hz; frequencies used in diagnostic ultrasound are much higher, typically between 2 and 18 MHz. The existence of ultrasound was recognized as early as the 18th century by Italian biologist Lazzaro Spallanzani, famous for his experiments on the navigation of bats flying in complete darkness. Bats, like dolphins, use ultrasound to map space and to locate sources of food.

Modern ultrasound technology is based on what is known as the *piezoelectric* effect, or the tendency of certain crystal or ceramic materials to produce electric current in response to mechanical pressure. Such materials are known as transducers, because they can transform energy. Pierre Curie was the first to identify this phenomenon. Together with his brother, Jacques, he demonstrated that compressing crystals such as quartz generated an electric current and that passing electric current through such crystals caused them to vibrate and emit sound waves. When the emitted sound bounced back to the transducing crystal, it in turn generated a current.

Directional sound reflections were initially applied for maritime use to detect objects and measure distances. Following the sinking of the *Titanic* in 1912, the Canadian R. A. Fessenden patented an early *sonar* (sound, navigation, and ranging) instrument capable of detecting icebergs within a two-mile range. Two years later, the threat of German submarines in World War I led French physicist and former Curie student Paul Langevin to develop an underwater sound generator, or hydrophone, to warn ships at sea of the proximity of large submerged objects. The first detection and subsequent sinking of a German U-boat using a hydrophone was recorded in early 1916. Langevin's ultrasound transducer is considered prototypical of modern ultrasound devices.

The piezoelectric principle eventually brought about the development of medical ultrasound, where the patient's body is explored by a transducer emitting and receiving sound waves reflected from various body structures. The transducer is connected to a computer, which transforms the signals received and sent by the ultrasound transducer into visual images. Early ultrasound equipment required cumbersome immersion of the patient's body. Technical advances have not only reduced the size of the apparatus, but have also made it portable. Handheld transducer probes generate and receive the ultrasonic waves. Their function is optimized by the use of aqueous gel applied to the patient's skin in order to eliminate any air that might reduce the transmission of the sound beam.

Medical applications of ultrasound were first investigated in the 1930s when the Viennese neurologist Karl Theodor Dussik attempted to produce ultrasonic images of the cerebral ventricles and locate brain tumors by holding transducers on either side of the skull. In the late 1940s U.S. naval officer George Ludwig described the localization of foreign bodies in animal tissue by means of pulse-echo ultrasound using an industrial metal flaw detector. Ludwig's experiments, in which he introduced a human gallstone in canine muscle and then attempted to locate it, are among the first to study acoustic impedance of different tissues.

At the same time Denver radiologist Douglas Howry, having first constructed an A-mode (amplitude mode) scanner, pioneered the two-dimensional B-mode (brightness mode) scanner. In the early 1950s, John J. Wild and John Reid at the University of Minnesota developed the first real-time handheld contact scanner. Their device, which consisted of a transducer enclosed in a water column sealed by a condom, could be swept manually over the examined tissue. Wild and Reid used this system to visualize breast cancer and other tumors, laying the foundation for noninvasive sonographic tissue diagnosis of mass lesions.

In 1953, Swedish researchers Inge Edler and Hellmuth Hertz expanded existing ultrasound modalities to include the imaging of heart structures. They developed the first echocardiographic image of a mitral valve. Their techniques were enhanced by the use of Doppler ultrasound, which employ the Doppler effect to characterize blood flow within the heart or the vascular system. Doppler ultrasound, named after 19th-century Austrian physicist Christian Doppler, measures the change in echo frequencies to calculate the speed of a moving object, and can thus measure the rate of blood flow. Nowadays, traditional M-mode (motion mode) echocardiography with added two-dimensional and Doppler scanning has become an essential tool in cardiac diagnosis, allowing the assessment not only of chamber size and pump function, but also the determination of valvular and myocardial integrity.

A key figure in 20th-century medical ultrasonography was Glasgow obstetrician-gynecologist Ian Donald. Donald, who confessed to an enduring "childish interest in machines, electronic and otherwise," had served in the Royal Air Force where he gained experience in sonar and radar (radio detection and ranging) techniques. He drew on Wild's work to investigate the medical use of industrial ultrasound equipment. First he conducted experiments on the ultrasonic characteristics of morbid anatomical specimens, then went on to evaluate pelvic tumors using a so-called "flaw detector" to distinguish solid from cystic growths. His 1958 landmark paper, *Investigation of Abdominal Masses by Pulsed Ultrasound*, published with John MacVicar and Tom Brown, would establish the incontrovertible diagnostic value of ultrasound.

Donald and his colleagues studied fetal growth and maturity, multiple pregnancy, and fetal anomalies. They made the first sonographic diagnosis of *placenta previa*, and in 1963 utilized the full bladder to detect very early stages of gestation. Initially limited to high-risk pregnancies, by the 1980s ultrasound had become standard in prenatal diagnosis.

Today, ultrasound is a routine part of medical care in the United States and many other countries. In children and adults alike, it is used to assess internal organs such as heart, liver, gallbladder, kidneys, breast, uterus, ovaries, and testes. Biliary and renal stones can be visualized, as can a full bladder, a dislocated hip, a ganglion cyst, or a deep venous clot. In obstetrical practice, the technique is used to follow fetal development in pregnancy, estimate delivery date, and determine gender of the child.

Increase in computing power has made possible "real-time" imaging, where changes in transducer position and internal anatomy are immediately reflected in the images produced. Compact and portable machines increasingly permit not only bedside but also emergency use. Ultrasound provides guidance in multiple procedures, such as guided tissue biopsies or placement of chest drainage tubes and central venous lines. So-called FAST (focused assessment with sonography in trauma) imaging can contribute to swift and timely treatment of intrathoracic and abdominal trauma.

Ultrasound testing is generally less expensive than other types of imaging, such as scanning by computed tomography (CT) or magnetic resonance (MR). Because it does not use ionizing radiation, it does not present any known health risks to the patient.

Bibliography and Suggested Readings

Gunderman, Richard B., *X-Ray Vision: The Evolution of Medical Imaging and Its Human Significance*, Oxford: Oxford University Press, 2013.

Kane, David, Grassi, Walter, Sturrock, Roger, and Balint, Peter V., "A Brief History of Musculoskeletal Ultrasound: 'From Bats and Ships to Babies and Hips'," *Rheumatology* 2004, 43(7): 931–933.

Kevles, Bettyann H., *Naked to the Bone: Medical Imaging in the Twentieth Century*, New Brunswick: Rutgers University Press, 1997.

Thomas, Adrian M. K., and Banerjee, Arpan K., *History of Radiology*, Oxford: Oxford University Press, 2013.

X-Rays

What	Electromagnetic waves capable of penetrating solid objects and substances. In medical radiography, the term refers to the image produced by positioning a part of the body in front of an X-ray detector and illuminating it with a short exposure. X-rays permit visualization of many inner structures and organs of the human body.
Where	Würzburg, Germany
When	1895
By Whom	Wilhelm Conrad Röntgen (1845–1923)
Importance	Major discovery that transformed the process of clinical diagnosis, especially in orthopedics and trauma medicine; led to the establishment of new medical specialties: diagnostic radiology and therapeutic radiology.

In November 1895, Wilhelm Röntgen, professor of physics at the University of Würzburg, discovered a previously unknown form of radiation. He had been investigating the phenomena produced by passing an electric current through a vacuum tube when he noticed that emissions from the tube were causing a faint glow on a nearby cardboard screen that had been painted with fluorescent barium platinocyanide. This glow persisted, even if he enclosed the discharge tube in thick black paper to block all light and operated in a completely darkened room. Moreover, the screen placed in the path of the rays became illuminated even when it was as far as two meters away from the tube.

What, other than visible light, could be causing the barium salts to fluoresce? Röntgen speculated that a new form of light might explain what he had observed, and for the next few weeks he devoted his time to investigating the nature of the new rays.

Subsequent experiments revealed that not only were the new rays able to migrate a distance beyond the tube, but also that they could travel through a variety of solid objects: a thick book, a piece of rubber, a wooden plank, or a sheet of aluminum; they did not penetrate certain other materials such as lead. Flesh appeared to be very translucent, whereas bones were fairly opaque. When Röntgen positioned his hand between the source of the rays and the piece of luminescent cardboard, he could see the bony skeleton of his living hand outlined upon the screen. Significantly, objects placed between the ray generator and a photographic plate produced "shadow pictures" on the plate. The investigator was thus able to make a permanent photographic record of the phenomena observed.

Two weeks following his initial experiment, Röntgen famously took the very first X-ray photograph of his wife Anna Bertha's hand. The developed plate showed the shadows thrown by the bones of her hand and by a ring she was wearing, all surrounded by the faint outline of her flesh more easily permeated by the rays. Otto Glasser, Röntgen's biographer, reports that when Frau Röntgen saw the skeletal outline of her hand she exclaimed: "I have seen my death!"

On December 28, 1895, Röntgen published his findings in a paper entitled *On a New Kind of Rays (Über eine neue Art von Strahlen)*. Because the nature of these rays was as yet unknown, he named them X-rays—after the mathematical designation X for an unknown factor. Soon thereafter news of his discovery appeared in the popular press, and scientists around the world began experimenting with the new rays. In 1896, only a few months after Röntgen's discovery, John Macintyre, a Scottish physician and former electrical engineer, set up the world's first radiology department at the Glasgow Royal Infirmary. There he produced the first X-ray of a kidney stone. In Birmingham the same year, Major Hall-Edwards became one of the first to use X-ray for the localization of a foreign body, discovering a needle embedded in a woman's hand; it was removed the following day.

Military doctors quickly saw the utility of the new technology. The British army installed X-ray machines in its London hospitals as early as 1896. The

Italian military was the first to use radiographs at the front, setting up X-ray–equipped field hospitals in East Africa during the first Abyssinian War. The British, too, transported field units to the front during the Nile campaign in Egypt, where, in the heat of the desert, soldiers were detailed to pedal bicycles reconstructed to activate portable electrical generators. Surgeon Francis Abbott described the challenges faced in treating wounded soldiers in the Greco-Turkish War and hailed the discovery of the Röntgen rays as "a new weapon [put] into the hands of the military surgeon." Battlefield injuries could now be assessed prior to treatment, and doctors were able to use mobile X-ray apparatus to detect bony fractures and hidden bullets.

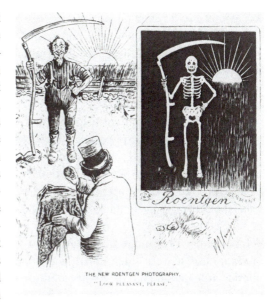

THE NEW ROENTGEN PHOTOGRAPHY.
"LOOK PLEASANT, PLEASE."

An 1896 *Life* magazine cartoon lampoons Wilhelm Röntgen's newly discovered X-rays. The 1895 invention was dismissed even by *The New York Times* as an "alleged discovery of how to photograph the invisible." In 1901, Röntgen was awarded the first Nobel Prize in Physics "in recognition for the extraordinary services rendered by . . . the remarkable rays." (AP Photo)

Among the public the new technology had generated a great deal of excitement from the very start. In some U.S. cities, department stores installed X-ray slot machines where, for a coin, customers could examine the bones of their own hands. In Paris, the wondrous new machines appeared together with public demonstrations of the Lumière brothers' new moving pictures. The American news baron William Randolph Hearst, in February 1896, commissioned Thomas Edison to produce a "cathodograph" of the human brain—a task that, however, proved impossible at the time.

Even as X-rays were shown to be a powerful diagnostic (and therapeutic) tool, the dangers of high-dose exposure to X-radiation were recognized. By the early 1900s many pioneering users had suffered severe burns. Francis Hall-Edwards's left arm had to be amputated in 1908. Edison's assistant, Clarence Dally, lost first his left hand, then both arms, and ultimately his life to the malignant ulcerations that had developed as a result of radiation dermatitis; he died in 1904. It took decades to set standards for permissible dosages and develop safety measures to protect workers, physicians, and patients alike from the harmful effects of excess radiation.

Wilhelm Röntgen had not been the first to produce X-rays. J. W. Hittorf (1824–1914), Sir William Crookes (1832–1919), Heinrich Hertz (1857–1894), Philipp von Lenard (1862–1947), and others had carried out previous experiments in this field. Their work defined many of the properties of the so-called cathode rays, an electric current established in highly rarefied gases by the high-tension electricity generated by an induction coil. But Röntgen—even though he himself was nearly blind in one eye as well as color-blind—was the first to detect the new rays and to understand their significance. He was widely honored for his discovery and, in 1901, was awarded the very first Nobel Prize in physics. Röntgen did not patent his findings, believing that they "belonged to mankind." He donated the money for his Nobel Prize—a sum today equivalent to $1.3 million—to his university.

The "invisible light" that Röntgen had discovered was a previously unknown type of electromagnetic radiation. Indeed, what we perceive as visible light is but a small fraction of the entire electromagnetic spectrum. X-rays—as German physicist Max von Laue showed a decade or so later with X-ray diffraction by crystals—are of the same electromagnetic nature as light, but differ from it in their shorter wavelength and in the higher frequency of their vibration.

Medical X-rays are generated by directing a stream of high-speed electrons at a target material, usually a metal plate such as tungsten, inside an X-ray tube; when the electrons are slowed or stopped by the target, X-radiation is produced. The shadow images produced by X-rays are due to the different absorption rates of individual body tissues. Calcium in bones has the highest absorption rate; therefore, bones appear white on an X-ray image or radiograph. Skin, fat, and connective and other soft tissues absorb less radiation and look gray. Air absorbs very little; consequently, air-inflated lung tissue or gas-containing bowel will look mostly black on X-ray.

The advent of X-rays transformed medical diagnostics. For the first time, physicians could probe the interior of the living body without cutting it open and visualize diseased and injured parts such as broken bones, foreign bodies, infections like pneumonia or internal abscesses, and other abnormal masses. Today X-rays are key in the diagnosis of fractures or other skeletal pathology. They are also standard in the evaluation of many soft tissue diseases. Plain chest films are commonly used to confirm pneumonia or congestive heart failure and to monitor their response to treatment. Abdominal plates can help define acute intra-abdominal problems such as intestinal obstruction or infection and biliary or renal stones.

The widespread use of X-rays led to the development of radiology, a new practice specialty made up of physicians and technologists trained in the interpretation of X-ray images and in the operation of complex imaging equipment. It is estimated that in the United States alone, over 30,000 radiologists and approximately 220,000 radiologic technologists are currently in active practice.

Bibliography and Suggested Readings

Gunderman, Richard B., *X-Ray Vision: The Evolution of Medical Imaging and Its Human Significance*, Oxford: Oxford University Press, 2013.

Howell, Joel, *Technology in the Hospital: Transforming Patient Care in the Early Twentieth Century,* Baltimore: Johns Hopkins University Press, 1995.

Kevles, Bettyann H., *Naked to the Bone: Medical Imaging in the Twentieth Century*, New Brunswick: Rutgers University Press, 1997.

Thomas, Adrian M. K., *The Invisible Light: 100 Years of Medical Radiology*, Oxford: Blackwell Science, 1995.

Thomas, Adrian M. K., and Banerjee, Arpan K., *History of Radiology*, Oxford: Oxford University Press, 2013.

Medications and Vaccines

Antihistamines

What	Compounds that block the effects of histamine, a biological substance released in allergic reactions, by binding to the body's histamine receptors.
Where	France; United Kingdom
When	1937–1941; 1972
By Whom	Daniel Bovet (1907–1992); James Black (1924–2010)
Importance	Essential first-line drugs for the treatment of allergic symptoms, including hay fever, hives, and itching; adjunctive treatment in asthmatic and anaphylactic syndromes.

For the millions of allergy sufferers worldwide, antihistamines have been life changing. Since their introduction in the 1940s they have become one of the most widely prescribed classes of drugs. As of 2015, antihistamines include two categories of drugs: the H1 histamine receptor antagonists and the H2 receptor antagonists. H1 antagonists are used in treating allergies of the upper respiratory tract (hay fever, rhinitis) and of the skin (hives, itching). They also help decrease severe allergic reactions and are adjuvants in the treatment of anaphylaxis. H2 antagonists reduce gastric acid secretion and are used in treating peptic ulcer disease and gastroesophageal reflux.

In medicinal chemistry, antihistamines were among the first "rational medicines": those intended to solve a specific biochemical problem by targeting the exact deficit or excess that produces the disease. Histamine, one of several substances released in the inflammatory process, had first been synthesized in 1907 from the naturally occurring amino acid histidine and was shown to play a critical role in immunological reactions. The task for physiological and pharmacological research was to find its antidote, or antagonist.

In 1902, French physiologist Charles Richet had demonstrated that animals could become sensitized to specific proteins after an initial contact or injection. Richet called this phenomenon *anaphylaxis* (as contrasted with *prophylaxis*).

Subsequent research showed that anaphylactic reactions could be induced not only by known poisonous substances but also by harmless ones. The reaction therefore depended not on a specific agent alone, but on some lasting alteration within the body, which upon subsequent exposure to this agent could induce potentially catastrophic adverse effects.

In 1902, Austrian physician Clemens von Pirquet observed a similar syndrome in patients who, after being given diphtheria antitoxin, developed fever, swelling, joint pains, itching, and widespread skin rash. Subsequent injections could lead to fulminant symptoms and even death. Called serum sickness, this was in fact an anaphylactic hypersensitivity reaction, resulting from a state of specific altered reactivity for which von Pirquet coined the term "allergy" (from the Greek *allos*, other, and *ergon*, action). Later studies demonstrated the relationship between anaphylaxis and hay fever, a chronic hypersensitivity condition caused by repeated exposure to environmental pollens. In susceptible individuals pollen functioned as the antigen that would, after a certain period of exposure, precipitate symptoms of hay fever.

Histamine was the first chemical to be identified as a likely contributor to allergic syndromes. When British physiologist Henry Dale and his collaborators set out to explore its biochemical action, they found that injecting it into experimental animals produced smooth muscle contraction and vasodilatation. Large doses produced effects similar to traumatic shock: constriction of the bronchial tree, fall in blood pressure and temperature, tachycardia, slowing of respirations, and altered mental status. Dale concluded that histamine played a major role in hypersensitivity reactions and that anaphylactic shock—a potentially fatal syndrome—was a result of cellular injury mediated by histamine.

Over the next few decades it was demonstrated that in shock, histamine-containing granules in mast cells released massive amounts of histamine, a prime mediator of the events observed. The physiological function of histamine is adjuvant because it helps the body remove inflammatory substances caused by cell damage. However, when histamine response is exaggerated, its effects lead to allergic disease or life-threatening anaphylaxis. Histamine is found in high concentrations in the skin and respiratory tract of allergic patients. Once circulating, it constricts the bronchi and relaxes vascular smooth muscle, which can lead to a precipitous fall in blood pressure. Histamine also increases capillary permeability, which leads to the escape of plasma proteins into the extravascular space and swelling of the surrounding tissues. These effects become manifest in the nasal congestion or itchy hives following contact with specific allergens.

The systematic search for a medicine that would block the effects of histamine and offer treatment for allergy began at the Pasteur Institute in Paris in the 1930s. It had long been recognized that one substance could counteract the physiological effects of another. This concept, just as that of an antidote to a poison, might equally apply to drugs if they were to be bound by a "receptive substance" in the body. Such a receptor, by combining with a specific drug, could then either initiate or inhibit physiological effects at the cellular level. Years earlier, Cambridge physiologist John Langley and German physician Paul Ehrlich had laid the foundations of the receptor theory of drug action. Together with the concept of drug specificity, receptor theory became a cornerstone of modern drug development.

The search for specific receptor antagonists to block histamine bore fruit in 1937 when a first antihistaminic compound was synthesized by Swiss pharmacologist Daniel Bovet and his collaborator Anne-Marie Staub. Too toxic, it was followed in 1941 by mepyramine, the first clinically usable antihistamine; it was marketed to the public as Neoantergan. Bovet's approach was based on his study of adrenergic and cholinergic antagonists and laid the foundation for effective synthesis of antihistamines. In 1942, French physician Bernard Halpern at the Rhône-Poulenc pharmaceutical laboratories developed Antergan, the first antihistamine to be patented in France. Others rapidly followed, including the still widely used diphenhydramine, developed in 1943 by American chemist George Rieveschl at the University of Cincinnati. Under its trade name Benadryl, this drug became synonymous with allergy relief.

By 1950, U.S. pharmaceutical companies would market more than 20 different antihistamines for conditions ranging from hives, hay fever, and eczema, to food and drug allergies. Antihistamines were also helpful in the treatment of minor transfusion reactions and allergy to IV contrast media in radiology. Off-label they were used as sedatives, sleeping aids, and antiemetics. In 1947, a combination of Benadryl and the bronchodilator theophylline was accidentally discovered to treat motion sickness, which led to the blockbuster drug Dramamine. After clinical testing on U.S. Army troops it was widely advertised as a cure for seasickness (*"The Drug that Makes Soldiers Good Sailors Will Soon Be Working for You!"*).

Now known as first-generation antihistamines, these early compounds were limited by their side effects, most commonly sedation, drowsiness, and drying of the mouth and mucous membranes. Development of the *second-generation*, nonsedating, antihistamines in the 1980s addressed these concerns. Designed to be chemically lipophobic, they did not penetrate the blood–brain barrier, and therefore had minimal effect on the patient's central nervous system and level of alertness. These newer compounds, including most recently cetirizine (Zyrtec), fexofenadine (Allegra), and loratadine (Claritin), have revolutionized the treatment of many widespread allergic conditions such as rhinitis, conjunctivitis, and urticaria.

In 1966, British pharmacologists showed that histamine receptors could be differentiated into at least two classes and proposed the name H1 receptors for those blocked by then-known antihistamines. In 1972, Scottish scientist James Black demonstrated the existence of a distinct group of H2 histamine receptors that mediate gastric acid secretion. He next synthesized a group of specific H2 blocking agents that ultimately led to the development of the H2 blocker cimetidine. Marketed as Tagamet, this compound was extremely effective in antagonizing the action of histamine in stimulating acid secretion and treating hypersecretory conditions. In 1986 the drug became the first ever to generate annual sales of more than $1 billion. Cimetidine not only relieved peptic ulcer symptoms and promoted healing in many patients, but also significantly decreased the need for surgical interventions. H2 blockers, although not curative, are still widely used in the treatment of disorders related to gastric acid production.

The identification of histamine and its antagonists were milestones in pharmacological and immunological research. They not only established the critical role of histamine in allergic disease and in gastric acid secretion, but also helped launch rational, targeted drug development. In 1957, the development of antihistamines active against H1 receptors earned Daniel Bovet a Nobel Prize in Physiology or Medicine; James Black, in turn, was awarded the 1988 Nobel Prize in Physiology or Medicine for discovering important drug treatment principles and identifying H2 receptors and their antagonists.

The discovery of antihistamines revolutionized treatment of histamine-mediated disease. In the industrialized world the prevalence of allergic diseases has continued to rise. Worldwide, allergic rhinitis alone affects between 10 and 30 percent of the population. In the United States, allergies are estimated to represent the sixth leading cause of chronic illness.

Bibliography and Suggested Readings

American Academy of Allergy, Asthma & Immunology, "Allergy Statistics," http://www.aaaai.org/about-the-aaaai/newsroom/allergy-statistics.aspx.

Emanuel, M. B., "Histamine and the Antiallergic Antihistamines: A History of Their Discoveries," *Clinical and Experimental Allergy* 1999, 29 (Suppl 3): 1–11.

Greaves, Malcolm W., "Antihistamines," *Dermatologic Clinics* January 2001, 19(1): 53–62.

Li, Jack, *Blockbuster Drugs: The Rise and Decline of the Pharmaceutical Industry*, Oxford: Oxford University Press, 2014.

Maehle, Andreas-Holger, " 'Receptive Substances': John Newport Langley (1852–1925) and His Path to a Receptor Theory of Drug Action," *Medical History* 2004, 48(2): 153–174.

Mitman, Greg, *Breathing Space: How Allergies Shape Our Lives and Landscapes*, New Haven: Yale University Press, 2008.

World Allergy Organization, http://www.worldallergy.org.

Aspirin

What	Aspirin, or acetylsalicylic acid (ASA), is a medication used primarily to relieve pain and reduce fever; it acts by inhibiting prostaglandins, which produce inflammation and sensitize pain receptors, and thromboxane, which is needed for blood clotting.
Where	England; France; Germany
When	1763; 1853; 1897; 1971
By Whom	Edmund Stone (1702–1768); Charles Gerhardt (1816–1856); Felix Hoffmann (1868–1946); John R. Vane (1927–2004)
Importance	Used to treat pain, fever, and inflammation; its blood-thinning properties make it essential in the prevention and treatment of heart attacks, strokes, and other vascular syndromes.

Aspirin was first produced commercially a little over 100 years ago and quickly became the most popular and successful synthetic medication worldwide. One of the oldest known drugs, its natural form, salicylic acid, is widely distributed throughout the plant kingdom. First identified in the leaves and bark of the willow, salicylate preparations had been used for thousands of years. Assyrians and Egyptians knew of the analgesic properties of willow extract, and the Ebers Papyrus (ca. 1543 BCE) described its application for joint pains and inflammatory conditions. In ancient Greece, Hippocrates recommended a decoction of willow leaves for relieving fevers and labor pains. Extracts of willow and myrtle for the treatment of inflammation, fever, and pain were widely used throughout the Roman Empire, as they were in North and Central America where native tribes made teas for medicinal use from the bark and twigs of the American white willow.

The English clergyman and scholar Edmund Stone is credited with the first scientific description of the beneficial effects of willow bark. In a 1763 letter to the Royal Society he reported preparing a powder from dried bark of the white willow tree to relieve fever and pain in more than 50 patients suffering from various "agues"—a term denoting intermittent fevers and pains, often symptomatic of malaria. He believed, as did many of his contemporaries, in the so-called doctrine of signatures according to which "like cures like." Hence, he had become interested in studying the healing properties of the willow, a plant flourishing in the same moist and wet conditions as many febrile illnesses. Reverend Stone likened the effects of willow bark to those of the much more costly Peruvian cinchona bark, the famous remedy containing quinine used to treat malaria.

An Account of the Success of the Bark of the Willow in the Cure of Agues. In a Letter to the Right Honourable George Earl of Macclesfield, President of R. S. from the Rev. Mr. Edmund Stone, of Chipping-Norton in Oxfordshire

Among the many useful discoveries which this age hath made . . . there is a bark of an English tree, which I have found by experience to be a powerful astringent, and very efficacious in curing aguish and intermitting disorders.

About six years ago, I accidentally tasted it, and was surprised at its extraordinary bitterness; which immediately raised me a suspicion of its having the properties of the Peruvian bark. As this tree delights in a moist or wet soil, where agues chiefly abound, the general maxim, that many natural maladies carry their cures along with them, or that their remedies lie not far from their causes, was so very apposite to this particular case, that I could not help applying it . . .

My curiosity prompted me to look into the dispensatories and books of botany, and examine what they said concerning it; but there it existed only by name. I could not find that it hath, or ever had, any place in pharmacy . . .

However, I determined to make some experiments with it; and, for this purpose, I gathered that summer near a pound weight of it, which I dried in a bag, upon the outside of a baker's oven, for more than three months, at which time it was to be reduced to a powder, by pounding and sifting . . .

It was not long before I had the opportunity of making a trial of it; but, being a stranger to its nature, I gave it in very small quantities . . . but with great caution and the strictest attention to its effects: the fits were considerably abated but did not entirely cease. Not perceiving the least ill consequences, I grew bolder with it, and in a few days increased the dose ... and the ague was soon removed.

It was then given to several others with the same success; but I found it better answered the intention when a dram of it was taken every four hours in the intervals of the paroxysms.

I have continued to use it as a remedy for agues and intermitting disorders for five years successively and successfully. It hath been given I believe to fifty persons, and never failed in the cure, except in a few ... agues ... [which] it reduced to a great degree ...

... [T]he patient was never prepared, either by vomiting, bleeding, purging, or any medicines of a similar intention, for the reception of this bark, ... and it was always given in powders with any common vehicle such as water, tea, small beer and such like. This was done purely to ascertain its effects; and that I might be assured the changes wrought in the patient could not be attributed to any other thing ...

The tree, from which this bark is taken, is ... the common white Willow.

Source: Edmund Stone, *Philosophical Transactions* 1763, 53: 195–200.

In the early 19th century, scientists, including Henri Leroux in France and Raffaele Piria in Italy, worked to isolate and purify the active ingredient of willow bark, salicin or salicylic acid (from the Latin *salix*, willow). Strasbourg chemist Charles Gerhardt in 1853 and Hermann Kolbe at Marburg in 1859 were the first to determine the molecular structure of the substance and synthesize a form of acetylsalicylic acid. This compound, with Leroux' and Piria's earlier sodium salicylate, became popular for the relief of pain and fever, but all had a number of negative side effects, most notably a painful irritation of the stomach.

In 1897 Felix Hoffmann, a young chemist working in the recently established pharmaceutical laboratory of German dye manufacturer Bayer in Elberfeld, succeeded in producing a chemically pure formulation that was not only stable but also better tolerated and more palatable. Hoffmann's research was undertaken at the reported direction of his colleague Arthur Eichengrün, and there has been historiographic controversy about who deserves credit for first synthesizing the compound. Recent re-examination of contemporary sources support Eichengrün's claim as well as the accusation of Nazi revisionism because Eichengrün was Jewish: he had been the one who instructed Hoffmann to synthesize acetylsalicylic acid using his own process, with the objective to obtain a drug that would not produce the frequent adverse effects of nausea, tinnitus, and gastric irritation associated with sodium salicylate. Eichengrün also secretly initiated early clinical trials against the directives of Heinrich Dreser, head of the pharmacology division, who believed the drug was harmful to the heart.

Ultimately, the compound was shown to have excellent results in inflammatory and rheumatic conditions, as well as in the treatment of pain and fever, with only rare tinnitus (ringing of the ears), and without unpleasant or deleterious effects on the stomach or the heart, even in very sick patients.

SAY "BAYER ASPIRIN" – *Genuine*

Unless you see the "Bayer Cross" on tablets, you are not getting the genuine Bayer Aspirin proved safe by millions and prescribed by physicians over 25 years.

DOES NOT AFFECT THE HEART

Safe → Accept only "Bayer" package which contains proven directions. Handy "Bayer" boxes of 12 tablets. Also bottles of 24 and 100—Druggists.

for Colds
Pain
Headache
Neuritis
Toothache
Neuralgia
Lumbago
Rheumatism

Aspirin is the trade mark of Bayer Manufacture of Monoaceticacidester of Salicylicacid

1920 advertisement urging consumers to "demand" the genuine, stamped Bayer product. The "drug of the century" quickly became a household word and the most popular painkiller worldwide. Contrary to the concern expressed in this ad, aspirin has now been shown to help prevent heart attacks and strokes. (AP Photo/Bayer)

In 1899 Bayer registered the new drug under the name "Aspirin" ("a" for acetyl, and "spir" for meadowsweet, *Spirea ulmaria*, a plant also rich in salicylates). The company sent information about the new drug to more than 30,000 physicians. It was the first mass marketing campaign of a pharmaceutical. Aspirin became not only Bayer's best-selling product but also the most popular drug of all time, in effect laying the foundation of the modern pharmaceutical industry. In 1904 the original powdered form was replaced with a stamped tablet so as to control dosing and prevent adulteration. The tablet became available as an "over-the-counter" medication, not requiring a prescription, in 1915. In 1950, aspirin was listed in the *Guinness Book of Records* as the most popular pain-killer in the world. Today it is estimated that more than 40,000 metric tons of aspirin are consumed worldwide every year.

Remarkably, it was not until 1971 that the mechanism of action of the world's most common drug was elucidated. This was when English pharmacologist John Vane reported that aspirin blocked the synthesis of hormonal mediators called prostaglandins and of thromboxane, a related substance. Prostaglandins, a group of inflammatory mediators formed from arachidonic acid, are released when cells undergo sudden changes due to stress, trauma, or disease. They are central in the development of inflammation—part of the body's natural healing process—producing fever, swelling, and painful sensory changes. Aspirin's anti-inflammatory effects are due to its suppression of the enzyme cyclooxygenase (COX), which converts arachidonic acid to prostaglandin. COX also plays a role in blood clotting and bleeding cessation by activation of thromboxane, a substance that causes platelets to clump together to facilitate the coagulation process. By interfering with the production of thromboxane, aspirin thins the blood by inhibiting platelet aggregation and clot formation; this explains how aspirin prevents thrombosis and reduces the risk of heart attacks and strokes. John Vane was awarded a Nobel Prize for his work in 1982.

Today, aspirin continues to be the most successful nonprescription medicine. In spite of occasional side effects, it remains a standard treatment for pain, fever, and inflammation. It is also one of the most investigated drugs; an estimated 1,000 clinical trials are conducted every year. Since the 1970s, numerous studies have shown its efficacy in reducing major cardiovascular events and in preventing heart attacks and strokes. Even dementia, probably of the multi-infarct type, is thought to benefit from long-term use of low-dose aspirin. Recent data analyses suggest that prophylactic use of aspirin may reduce the incidence of bowel, gastric, and esophageal cancers.

Bibliography and Suggested Readings

Cusick, Jack, et al., "Estimates of Benefits and Harms of Prophylactic Use of Aspirin in the General Population," *Annals of Oncology* 2015, 26(1): 47–57.

Elwood, Peter, "Aspirin, Past, Present, and Future," *Clinical Medicine* March/April 2001, 1(2): 132–137.

Jack, David B., "One Hundred Years of Aspirin," *Lancet* 1997, 350(9075): 437–439.

Jeffreys, Diarmuid, *Aspirin, the Remarkable Story of a Wonder Drug*, London: Bloomsbury, 2004.

Sneader, Walter, "The Discovery of Aspirin: A Reappraisal," *British Medical Journal* December 2000, 321(7276): 1591–1594.

Birth Control Pill

What	A medication taken by mouth to prevent pregnancy; known as birth control pill, or oral contraceptive (OCP), it acts by inhibiting ovulation. OCPs usually consist of a combination of synthetic progesterone and estrogen, the two major female sex hormones.
Where	Austria; Mexico; United States
When	1921; 1951; 1955; 1960
By Whom	Ludwig Haberlandt (1885–1932); Carl Djerassi (b.1923); Gregory Pincus (1903–1967); John Rock (1890–1984); Margaret Sanger (1879–1966)
Importance	Transformed the life of millions of women, couples, and families by making possible reproductive control.

On May 9, 1960, the U.S. Food and Drug Administration (FDA) approved the world's first birth control pill. The radically new method allowed couples for the first time to separate procreation from the sexual act, did not require male cooperation, and was nearly 100 percent effective in preventing pregnancy. The "Pill" not only revolutionized birth control but also initiated broad debate on a subject heretofore taboo in many circles.

As early as 1921, Austrian physiologist Ludwig Haberlandt had shown that sex hormones could suppress ovulation in animals. After implanting the ovaries of a pregnant rabbit into another, the recipient animal remained infertile for several months. In 1930 Haberlandt confirmed successful experiments in mice with an orally administered hormonal preparation, "Infecundin," which induced temporary infertility. His 1931 treatise on the subject concluded that "practical application of temporary hormonal sterilization in women" might turn into reality a longstanding ideal in human society, namely "the elevation of procreation into a voluntary and deliberate act." Haberlandt's views on reproductive biology and contraception ran afoul of the political, moral, and religious views of the time, and his colleagues accused him of hindering unborn life. In 1932, at the age of 47 and at the peak of his scientific career, the "grandfather of the Pill" committed suicide. His work fell into oblivion until 1966, when "Infecundin" became the trade name of the first oral contraceptive manufactured in Hungary.

Within a few years of Haberlandt's research, other scientists in Europe and the United States demonstrated that high doses of estrogens and progesterone could inhibit ovulation in animals. However, synthesizing clinically useful progesterone from naturally occurring steroid precursors (mostly cholesterol and bile acids) was a complex process, which limited production and made the substance very expensive. This changed in the early 1940s, when Pennsylvania chemistry professor Russell Marker discovered a method of synthesizing progesterone from a naturally occurring, inexpensive plant source in diosgenin, a component of the wild Mexican yam. Unable to find commercial sponsorship in the United States, he moved to Mexico City and continued his work with a small local laboratory, later to become *Syntex*; together they made production of progesterone commercially viable. By 1950 Marker's process had become the cornerstone of a large-scale Mexican steroid industry supplying hormones such as cortisone and testosterone to pharmaceutical companies worldwide.

None of the early synthetic progesterones could be taken by mouth, because they did not resist enzymatic breakdown in the digestive tract. In 1951, American chemist Carl Djerassi succeeded in producing an analog that had both greater progestational potency and oral efficacy. His compound, a modified testosterone molecule called "norethindrone," was the first oral contraceptive to be synthesized. The chemistry of the Pill had been conceived.

Neither Djerassi nor his collaborators were interested in contraception when they developed an oral progestin; they were trying to find a drug for treating menstrual disorders and infertility. It was biochemist Gregory Pincus, director of the Worcester Foundation for Experimental Biology, who pursued the anti-ovulatory effects of progesterone. Pincus' research was supported early on by New York nurse and birth control pioneer Margaret Sanger. An ardent feminist who had herself witnessed the consequences of unwanted pregnancies (her own mother had 18 pregnancies), Sanger had opened the first U.S. birth control clinic in 1916. In 1951, she asked Pincus to investigate hormonal contraception, ideally as a pill that would be "harmless, reliable, practical, universally applicable, and . . . satisfactory to both husband and wife." Up until then, the only available contraceptives were barrier devices, such as condoms, sponges, and diaphragms, or postcoital douches; other practices included withdrawal prior to ejaculation, calendar-based rhythm methods, or periodic abstinence. None were reliably effective or very practical. Moreover, contraceptive devices were illegal in the United States and Europe; in the United States, the 1873 Comstock Act had banned all materials relating to sex education and contraception as obscene and immoral. Sanger's idea of a pregnancy-preventing pill for women was thus controversial in many quarters, but it was supported and largely funded by her friend, the activist heiress and philanthropist Katharine McCormick who, like Sanger, saw reproductive control as essential to women's emancipation and self-determination.

Excerpts from Margaret Sanger's 1928 "Motherhood in Bondage," a collection of 470 letters selected from the many thousands she received, asking for help and pleading for information about birth control.

Section 1, Girl Mothers

Two

The reason I send for information is because I think if any woman needs help I am the one. I am seventeen years old. I married when I was thirteen and I am the mother of six children. My first baby was thirteen months old when another was born, then ten months after that I had twins and ten months later another set of twins. Now I am to have some more. My husband gets awful cross with me when I get this way, because, like you say in your book, he thinks we have got plenty. It is also wearing me down. I never feel well.

Section 3, The Trap of Maternity

Five

I am the mother of nineteen children, the baby only 20 months old. I am forty-three years old and I had rather die than give birth to another child. The doctor does not give me any information at all, only to be careful. This letter may sound unreasonable, but the records will show that it is true. I have five boys and seven girls living. Two daughters married. One has four children and the other one has five daughters. Have bad health. I need the information for them as well as myself, so for my sake and for the sake of humanity please give me the proper information.

Nine

I have tried so hard not to become pregnant but now I am pregnant again after having given birth to fourteen children. It seems to me it was more than one woman should be asked to. It sure makes my heart and hands full. Husband has cancer of the stomach and I have wanted to be all the comfort to him possible but now my heart is broken and makes me feel like giving up. The oldest child is twenty-four and my last baby was three and now I am along three months again. What should a woman do? It sure seems like a woman should have a limited number of children. I love babies but how can one do justice to a little bunch like this. I some times do not see how I ever have stood it all. I don't see why the law should not be in favor of contraceptives, unless it is that it is in a man's hands and he does not have to suffer the consequences.

Section 11, The Husband's Own Story

Eleven

My wife cannot carry pregnancy through to birth. She has had to be aborted twice "according to law" in order to save her life. This has ruined her health and almost destroyed our home. The doctors and hospitals are very willing to make big charges for these operations, but will not give any information regarding the prevention of pregnancy, although they say it must not happen again. Her condition of course makes conception doubly easy. I am trying to protect her by practicing continence. But this is not desirable nor good for either of us. I am a poor man working on a salary. My wife is very timid and backward about seeking information, so I am presuming to write to you myself, as I want to protect her and save our home.

Source: Margaret Sanger, *Motherhood in Bondage*, New York: Brentanos, 1928. Used by permission of Alexander Sanger.

Pincus' studies soon confirmed that progesterone inhibited ovulation in rabbits and rats. At the same time, Harvard gynecologist John Rock, an expert in fertility disorders, was experimenting with oral administration of estrogen and progesterone to treat infertile women. He found that high doses of sex steroids promoted uterine growth and could restore fertility; the very same treatment also suppressed ovulation.

In 1954 Pincus and Rock joined forces to develop an oral contraceptive. Among the many substances they tested, the two most promising were Djerassi's norethindrone and its isomer, norethynodrel, developed in 1952 by Frank Colton; they eventually selected this compound, produced by the Searle Company of Chicago, for their experimental trials.

Under the guise of an infertility study, John Rock—a Catholic who challenged his church on the subject of contraception—conducted a successful early trial of the Searle pill in 50 Boston women. Progesterone was administered for 21 days, followed by a 7-day break to allow for menstruation, so as to mimic the natural menstrual cycle and hopefully stave off controversy: such a rhythm-like method might be held morally acceptable by the Vatican because it simply extended women's "safe" period. Nevertheless, large-scale clinical trials necessary for FDA approval could not be carried out in Massachusetts because of legal constraints. Rock and Pincus, therefore, in 1956, initiated a large clinical trial of norethynodrel in Puerto Rico where no anticontraceptive prohibitions existed, enrolling over 200 women from a San Juan housing project in their study. Some of their pills had been contaminated with a small amount of synthetic estrogen but turned out to cause less breakthrough bleeding than the purified form. As a result, the final experimental drug was formulated to contain a tiny amount of estrogen in addition to the progesterone, a combination still used today.

Their study results were conclusive, and news of a contraceptive pill giving "100 percent protection against pregnancy" quickly spread. In 1957, the FDA approved the first contraceptive pill, Enovid, for the treatment of severe menstrual disorders, with the warning that the drug would prevent ovulation. Soon after FDA approval, unusual numbers of American women developed severe menstrual disorders and asked their doctors for the pill, presumably for off-label contraceptive purposes. In 1960 the FDA broadened Enovid's approved indications to include contraception. Clinical trials in other countries followed, eventually leading to refined dosages and hormonal components of the initial contraceptive.

Inhibition of ovulation was the primary mechanism of action of the Pill; animal studies and synthesis of orally active sex steroids had been its necessary underpinnings. It was a small miracle that the drug could be introduced before the complex endocrinology of ovulation and the menstrual cycle was fully understood. Another major obstacle in its development was the prevailing anticontraceptive climate of the time. Social forces; the feminist movement; and the determination of women such as Sanger, McCormick, and others like Estelle Griswold, Connecticut Director of Planned Parenthood, were instrumental in overcoming these obstacles. Starting in 1965, the U.S. Supreme Court issued a series of rulings overturning state laws banning contraception. In *Griswold v. Connecticut*, the Court held that prohibition of contraceptives was unconstitutional because it violated a married couple's right to privacy; this ruling was later extended to include nonmarried couples. Abroad, Catholic countries such as France, Spain, and Italy gradually eliminated their bans on birth control, although in Ireland contraceptives remained illegal until 1980. The Vatican to this day continues to condemn use of the Pill; Pope Paul VI in his 1968 encyclical *Humanae Vitae* designated it an artificial and therefore sinful method that might easily lead toward conjugal infidelity and low morals. Across the world, however, women welcomed the new contraceptive. Millions were using it within just a few years.

Soon after the Pill's introduction, potential life-threatening side effects such as blood clots and strokes became a concern. By the late sixties, it was clear that cardiovascular risk was directly related to estrogen dosage and that the Pill was equally effective with lower amounts of estrogen. Current research deems oral contraceptives to be safe for use in most women and to present fewer risks than those associated with pregnancy. The combination progesterone-estrogen pill also has noncontraceptive and therapeutic benefits: it can protect against ovarian and uterine cancers, as well as treat other disorders such as menorrhagia, acne, and hirsutism.

Over the years, social and moral objections to birth control have faded, so that most would consider the advent of reliable oral contraception a major achievement of modern medical science. For millions of men and women, but especially for women, the Pill relieved the fears of unwanted pregnancy. It prevented untold deaths from illegal abortion or childbirth, and it allowed many thousands of women to develop their personal and professional lives unhampered by untimely childbearing. Today, the Pill is the most common method of contraception in the Western world, used by over 100 million women.

Bibliography and Suggested Readings

Dhont, Marc, "History of Oral Contraception," *European Journal of Contraception and Reproductive Health Care* December 2010, 15(2): 12–18.

Eig, Jonathan, *The Birth of the Pill: How Four Crusaders Reinvented Sex and Launched a Revolution*, New York: W.W. Norton, 2014.

Junod, Suzanne W., and Marks, Lara, "Women's Trials: The Approval of the First Oral Contraceptive Pill in the United States and Great Britain," *Journal of the History of Medicine and Allied Sciences* 2002, 57(2): 117–160.

Liao, Pamela Verma, and Dollin, Janet, "Half a Century of the Oral Contraceptive Pill: Historical Review and View to the Future," *Canadian Family Physician* 2012, 58(12): 757–760.

Marsh, Margaret, and Ronner, Wanda, *The Fertility Doctor: John Rock and the Reproductive Revolution*, Baltimore: Johns Hopkins University Press, 2008.

May, Elaine Tyler, *America and the Pill: A History of Promise, Peril, and Liberation*, New York: Basic Books, 2010.

Chemotherapy

What	The use of chemical compounds to treat and cure cancer.
Where	United States
When	1940s; 1950s, and ongoing
By Whom	Sidney Farber (1903–1973); Alfred Gilman (1908–1984); Louis Goodman (1906–2000); Min Chiu Li (1919–1980); many others
Importance	Dramatically affected treatment and survival of cancer patients.

Cancer, an ancient disease, remains one of the most feared. Its causes were long mysterious and its cure elusive. Scientific innovations delivered clean water, aseptic surgery, and miracle drugs, but until the 1950s cancer had not been amenable to such medical progress. Treatment consisted of surgical extirpation or radiotherapy and was often unsuccessful or merely palliative. But starting in 1948, new cancer chemotherapies began to affect survival of cancer patients and transform patient expectations of cure.

The idea that chemicals could cure cancer was revolutionary. Animal experiments had shown that certain physical or chemical agents, including radioactive substances, ultraviolet light, and X-rays, could induce cancerous changes at the cellular level. Nobel laureate Paul Ehrlich in the early 20th century was the first to try "chemotherapy," the systematic targeting of cancer cells with chemical compounds. Following his lead, scientists started screening for effective cancer drugs using transplantable tumors in laboratory animals.

The use of chemical weapons in World War I had stimulated a great deal of research on sulfur mustard, a vesicant and deadly poison gas. The highly toxic substance not only burnt and blistered the skin and mucous membranes of exposed victims, but also depleted their cell-forming bone marrow. In the late 1930s while investigating the therapeutic use of mustard compounds, Yale pharmacologists Alfred Gilman and Louis Goodman discovered that substituting a nitrogen for the sulfur atom resulted in a less toxic substance. This had antitumor activity in mouse lymphoma. Administration of nitrogen mustard resulted not only in marked depletion of normal white cells, but also in regression of transplanted lymphoid tumors.

The discovery led the two researchers to focus on lymph gland cancers, or lymphomas, in human patients. In 1942, their experimental infusion of intravenous nitrogen mustard achieved temporary remission in a 48-year-old man with severe airway obstruction from swollen lymphoid tissue. Marked, albeit temporary, regression was also observed in other lymphoma patients.

Wartime secrecy regarding use of poison gases, heightened by the tragic spill of a secret Allied cargo of mustard gas in the Italian harbor of Bari, precluded early release of these reports. When Gilman and Goodman's findings were finally published in 1946, they sparked a flurry of research into compounds related to nitrogen mustard. Chlorambucil and cyclophosphamide, important less toxic oral derivatives, were developed in the 1950s.

Meanwhile, in Boston, pathologist Sidney Farber conducted parallel investigations centering on folate antagonists. Nutritional studies in the late 1930s and early 1940s had shown that green leafy vegetables were essential for normal bone marrow function. A key ingredient was folic acid, first synthesized in 1937. Its deficiency produced a bone marrow depletion similar to that induced by exposure to nitrogen mustard. Farber was first to test the role of folic acid in acute childhood leukemia, a bone marrow cancer causing proliferation of malignant white blood cells and depletion of the other marrow constituents: red cells and platelets. This disease was invariably and rapidly fatal.

Farber quickly discovered that using folic acid actually accelerated abnormal cell growth and worsened leukemia. He therefore tried a series of folate antagonists, including aminopterin and amethopterin (now known as methotrexate) synthesized by biochemist Yellapragada Subbarao. These compounds induced clear-cut suppression of cancer cell production and temporary remission in Farber's young leukemia patients. Methotrexate has proved to be effective for a number of cancers. It is still used either alone or in combination with other agents for the treatment of leukemia, lymphoma, and various other neoplasms, including cancers of the head and neck, lung, and breast.

In 1948, the same time methotrexate was first used in childhood leukemia, U.S. chemists George Hitchings and Gertrude Elion isolated the antimetabolite that led to the development of 6-thioguanine and 6-mercaptopurine. These compounds were structural analogs of natural purines and blocked DNA production. They became widely used in acute leukemia and certain viral infections and for immunosuppression in organ transplantation. Hitchings and Elion were awarded the 1988 Nobel Prize in Physiology or Medicine for their discovery.

Another important chemotherapeutic agent, 5-fluorouracil (5-FU), stemmed from the research of Charles Heidelberger, a biochemist at the University of Wisconsin. He had recognized that in certain cancers there was abnormal uptake and metabolism of uracil, one of the pyrimidine nucleic acids of RNA; his compound specifically targeted this biochemical pathway. 5-FU was found to have broad activity against solid tumors and remains to this day a key adjuvant in the treatment of colorectal cancer.

Antibiotics, too, were examined for potential antitumor activity, leading to the isolation of actinomycin D from a soil bacterium; used together with radiation it induced remission in Wilms's tumor, a rare form of kidney cancer in children. Today, actinomycin D is included in the list of essential medicines published by the World Health Organization and treats a variety of cancers.

These discoveries marked a turning point in cancer treatment and transformed American cancer research. In 1955, helped by the indefatigable Farber champion and philanthropist Mary Lasker, the Cancer Chemotherapy National Service Center (CCNSC) was established within the National Cancer Institute (NCI). Its mission was to support pharmacological research and testing. Fifteen years later, passage of the National Cancer Act in 1971 gave the NCI unprecedented autonomy and public funding and launched President Richard Nixon's "War Against Cancer."

Still, efforts to develop cancer chemotherapy remained controversial, not least because of the drugs' many toxic side effects. Moreover, although dramatic clinical remissions had been achieved, they were often only temporary and not curative. When NCI physician Min Chiu Li in 1958 reported that systemic chemotherapy could cure choriocarcinoma, a rare tumor of the placenta, it was a breakthrough that most of his contemporaries were not prepared to recognize. Using high doses of methotrexate for several days and titrating treatment to patients' level of hCG (human chorionic gonadotropin) hormone, Li had achieved complete remission in three cases of metastatic disease.

This became a new but essential principle in cancer treatment. Li had in effect identified a biochemical "tumor marker," the presence of which indicated that cancer recurrence was likely. Choriocarcinoma, usually fatal within a year of diagnosis, is today nearly always curable with chemotherapy.

In 1960 Li also developed the first successful multidrug chemotherapy for the treatment of metastatic testicular cancer. His combination regimen has virtually eliminated deaths as a result of this malignancy.

Other advances followed, including discovery of the cytotoxic activity of the periwinkle plant, or *Vinca rosea*. Vinca alkaloids such as vincristine and vinblastine arrest cell division. A regimen known as "VAMP" (vincristine, amethopterin, 6-mercaptopurine, and prednisone) proved to be superior to single agents: the combination increased rates and duration of remissions in leukemia by years, effectively leading to cure.

The notion of cure was a breakthrough for the use of anticancer drugs and helped overcome much of the medical pessimism prevailing in the 1960s and 1970s. Today, thanks to chemotherapy, the vast majority of children with acute lymphoblastic leukemia are cured, as are 90 percent of adult patients with advanced Hodgkin's lymphoma. A number of solid tumors in adults are also treatable.

In addition, largely due to the work of Pennsylvania surgeon Bernard Fisher, adjuvant chemotherapy (the use of drugs as adjuncts to surgery or radiotherapy) was established as beneficial, especially in early-stage breast cancer. Fighting possible occult metastases by treating earlier localized cancers with adjuvants to surgery has become the norm and has contributed to a significant decline in breast and colorectal cancer mortality.

Cancer, we now know, is caused by uncontrolled replication of cells, where normal regulatory mechanisms of cell division and cell death have gone awry. Underlying this uncontrolled malignant growth are genetic mutations. As our knowledge of these mutations has evolved, so has our search for better drugs and more specific, less toxic, treatments. Today, new immune cell therapies try to harness the natural defenses of our immune system. Monoclonal antibodies are engineered to target abnormal cells for destruction. Some immunotherapies used in conjunction with traditional chemotherapy have already proved successful.

The discovery that combinations of cytotoxic chemicals could cure certain cancers ranks among the major advances of 20th-century medicine. Since the 1970s, along with the establishment of the field of medical oncology, cancer treatment programs have grown exponentially. In the United States the budget allocated to wage the cancer war has ballooned 25-fold, from $220 million in 1971 to $5.1 billion in 2011, and spawned a multibillion-dollar pharmaceutical industry. Cancer mortality since 1990, in spite of a larger and aging population, has steadily declined. Although much of this decline is due to preventive efforts and earlier detection, much is also the result of modern chemotherapy as an integral part of cancer treatment.

Bibliography and Suggested Readings

American Cancer Society, "The History of Cancer," http://www.cancer.org/cancer/cancerbasics/thehistoryofcancer/index.

DeVita Jr., Vincent, and Chu, Edward, "A History of Cancer Chemotherapy," *Cancer Research* 2008, 68(21): 8643–8653.

Galmarini, Darío, et al., "Cancer Chemotherapy: A Critical Analysis of Its 60 Years of History," *Critical Reviews in Oncology and Hematology* 2012, 84(2): 181–199.

Morrison, Wallace B., "Cancer Chemotherapy: An Annotated History," *Journal of Veterinary Internal Medicine* 2010, 24(6): 1249–1262.

Mukherjee, Siddhartha, *The Emperor of All Maladies: A Biography of Cancer*, New York: Scribner, 2010.

Cortisone

What	A steroid hormone produced by the cortex of the adrenal gland and released in response to stress. Together with adrenaline, cortisone raises blood pressure and prepares the body for a "fight or flight" reaction.
Where	United States; Switzerland
When	1935; 1948
By Whom	Edward Calvin Kendall (1886–1972); Tadeus Reichstein (1897–1996); Philip Showalter Hench (1896–1965)
Importance	Vital medicinal uses in the treatment of inflammatory diseases such as arthritis and asthma; reduces local pain and inflammation.

Cortisone, an organic hydrocarbon compound of the steroid family, was first isolated from the adrenal cortex in 1935 by Edward Kendall at the Mayo Clinic and Tadeus Reichstein at the University of Basel. It has since become one of the most important therapeutic agents in modern medicine.

For a long time little was known about the function of the adrenal glands, the two small organs located at the upper poles of the kidneys. These ductless endocrine glands consist of two distinct anatomical parts: an outer firm shell, or cortex, and an inner soft center, or medulla. The 19th-century English physician Thomas Addison was the first to show that destruction of the adrenal glands led to anemia, severe fatigue, weakness of the heart, and a characteristic bronze pigmentation of the skin—hallmarks of what is now known as Addison's disease. This condition was uniformly fatal.

Addison's findings stimulated efforts to identify the active substance necessary to prevent adrenal disease. In 1934 Edward Kendall at the Mayo Clinic in Rochester, Minnesota, succeeded in producing a mixture of so-called "cortins." These substances all belonged to the important group of steroid hormones. Their structure resembled that of the male sex hormone, as well as of D vitamins and bile acids. Distinguishing between these chemically analogous substances was challenging, because they exist in the cortex in only small quantities and quickly form mixed crystals. At least six of these cortins, however, proved to have an effect on animals whose adrenals had been removed. Kendall and Reichstein were the first to identify them. Cortisone, or Compound E as Kendall had first named it, best known of all the active cortin substances, was isolated at both laboratories.

Initially, cortisone was not used in clinical medicine because the yield of tissue extractions was extremely low, less than 100 mg per 100 lbs of adrenal glands. The impetus to develop better production methods came in the early 1940s. Rumors that German pilots were taking adrenal extracts to combat altitude sickness spurred the pursuit of large-scale hormone production for possible strategic use during World War II. In 1944 Merck chemist Lewis Sarrett developed the first synthetic cortisone by extracting minute quantities of the hormone from ox bile. However, his method entailed a lengthy multistep process resulting in a final yield of only 0.01 percent. This meant that in order to treat one patient for one year approximately 14,000 cows would have to be slaughtered! The cost of an ounce of cortisone was exorbitant, and by 1948 Merck had produced only about 10 grams.

It was a portion of this precious supply that was shipped to the Mayo Clinic in 1948 for clinical testing by physician Philip Hench. Hench, an early rheumatologist and long-time collaborator of Kendall, had noted that in pregnancy and in cases of jaundice, rheumatic illness often improved. He theorized that this might be due to a common metabolic factor linked to adrenal function. Indeed, sex hormone and bile acid levels respectively increase in these conditions; both are related to cortin substances. Hench had previously experimented with cortins to treat rheumatoid arthritis, a debilitating inflammatory joint disorder. When cortisone became available, he tested it on a young woman afflicted by the crippling disease. Until then she had been refractory to all therapeutic trials. Two of his colleagues injected the patient with 100 mg of Kendall's "Compound E" (cortisone). The results were spectacular. Her dramatic improvement allowed reduction of daily dosing to 25 mg within three days, and Kendall reported that within a week "she walked out of the hospital in a gay mood and went on a shopping trip . . ."

Similar successes were achieved in several other patients over the following months. Their joint pain and swelling improved rapidly, and bedridden sufferers were able to walk again. Unfortunately, when the limited supplies ran out, all of them relapsed. Nevertheless, an important scientific breakthrough had been achieved.

Kendall and Hench published their findings in early 1949. Soon widely confirmed by others, they ushered in a new era in the treatment of inflammatory diseases. Cortisone was hailed as a miracle drug, and together with penicillin and streptomycin epitomized the major therapeutic advances of the 20th century. In 1950, only a year later, Hench, Kendall, and Reichstein were jointly awarded the Nobel Prize in Physiology or Medicine in recognition of their work.

In those early days cortisone was in tight supply. In the United Kingdom, strict policies limited its distribution exclusively to approved research units. In the United States, a free market developed in which cortisone initially sold for as much as $1,000 per gram. Many patients came to believe that higher doses of the drug would provide even better relief. As a consequence, some of them became dependent on the medication and had to obtain it on the black market or offer themselves as study subjects for invasive experiments.

Over the following decade, the process of cortisone synthesis was simplified. In the 1950s diosgenin, a substance extracted from the Mexican wild yam, replaced bovine bile acid as source material for the industrial production of a number of steroid hormones. This not only made production of cortisone commercially viable, but also greatly reduced its cost. In recent years the development of genetically engineered microorganisms has made possible the total biosynthesis of cortisone.

Today, cortisone and its analogs remain among the most commonly prescribed medications and are used in the treatment of a variety of inflammatory conditions. Corticosteroids are essential for treating severe allergic reactions, asthma, burns, and traumatic brain injuries. They also have an important role in transplant medicine, where they help to suppress the body's immune system and prevent transplant rejection. Long-term cortisone treatment, however, can result in a number of adverse side effects, including weight gain, hypertension, diabetes, osteoporosis, hair and skin changes, and increased susceptibility to infection.

A milestone in modern medicine, the discovery of cortisone contributed to the development of endocrinology and rheumatology as medical disciplines.

Bibliography and Suggested Readings

Glyn, John, "The Discovery and Early Use of Cortisone," *Journal of the Royal Society of Medicine* October 1998, 91: 513–517.

Hench, Philip S., "The Reversibility of Certain Rheumatic and Non-Rheumatic Conditions by the Use of Cortisone or of the Pituitary Adrenocorticotropic Hormone," *Nobel Lectures, Physiology or Medicine, 1942–1962*, Amsterdam: Elsevier Publishing Company, 1964, pp. 312–341.

Hillier, Stephen G., "Diamonds Are Forever: The Cortisone Legacy," *Journal of Endocrinology* October 2007, 195(1): 1–6.

Kendall, Edward C., "The Development of Cortisone as a Therapeutic Agent," *Nobel Lectures, Physiology or Medicine, 1942–1962,* Amsterdam: Elsevier, 1964, pp. 270–288.

Kendall, Edward C., "Hormones of the Adrenal Cortex in Health and Disease," *Proceedings of the American Philosophical Society* 1953, 97: 8–11.

Werth, Barry, *The Billion-Dollar Molecule: One Company's Quest for the Perfect Drug*, New York: Simon & Schuster, 1994.

Diphtheria Toxoid

What	Vaccine made of formalin-inactivated diphtheria toxin that provides active acquired immunity against diphtheria.
Where	Germany; France; England
When	1890; 1922
By Whom	Emil Behring (1854–1917); Paul Ehrlich (1954–1915); Gaston Ramon (1886–1963); Alexander Thomas Glenny (1882–1965)
Importance	Major advance in immunology and infectious disease prevention; first introduction of serum therapy and passive immunization; toxoid vaccines revolutionized approach to vaccination.

Diphtheria was a major cause of childhood death until the early 20th century. The isolation of *Corynebacterium diphtheriae* and that of the toxin secreted by the organism were pioneering discoveries. In the 1920s diphtheria toxoid was introduced for mass immunization, ultimately leading to control of the disease.

Diphtheria had been described as far back as Babylonian and Sumerian times. Known as the "strangling angel of children," classical diphtheria (from the Greek for "leather," denoting the tough membrane coating the throat) infects the upper respiratory tract with symptoms of sore throat and fever that progress to airway obstruction. In severe cases, swelling of the soft tissues of the neck and formation of a pseudo-membrane, a thick gray or yellowish coating of the pharynx, lead to complete blockage of the air passages resulting in suffocation and death. The diphtheria toxin first causes damage to local capillaries and eventually affects distant organs, especially the heart muscle and nervous system; the majority of patients with severe infection develop neurological complications, including paralysis of the soft palate and pharynx, as well as of eye and facial muscles.

The disease seems to have originated in the Middle East, from where it spread to Europe and other continents. Epidemic outbreaks often occurred in times of war. In the early 19th century diphtheria became a leading cause of infant mortality, with death rates as high as 80 percent; it was often associated with poverty, overcrowding, and poor nutrition in urban populations. At that time, treatments were limited to mechanical interventions such as tracheostomy, introduced in 1825 by French physician Pierre Bretonneau, and airway intubation, introduced by Eugène Bouchut in 1858. Bretonneau named the infection and detailed its clinical features, including the appearance of the pathognomonic pseudo-membrane.

In 1883, German pathologist Edwin Klebs first described the diphtheria bacillus. The following year bacteriologist Friedrich Loeffler grew it in pure culture. Both Klebs and Loeffler demonstrated a causal relationship between the bacillus and the membranous pharyngitis, showing that cultures caused disease in test animals in accordance with Koch's famous postulates. Having observed that *C. diphtheriae* colonized the nasopharynx but did not invade deeper parts of the body, Loeffler, in 1884, postulated the existence of another highly poisonous substance responsible for the lethal injury to respiratory and other organs. Four years later, Pasteur scientists Emile Roux and Alexandre Yersin confirmed Loeffler's hypothesis: they observed that after injection of bacteria-free filtrates of *C. diphtheriae* cultures, animals developed tissue damage indistinguishable from that seen in human diphtheria cases, thus demonstrating that there was indeed a lethal toxin to account for disease fatality.

Diphtheria toxin, so deadly in the infection, was also key in its successful treatment and prevention. As early as 1890, Emil Behring and Shibasaburo Kitasato investigated the use of "antitoxin" (a term they coined) in convalescent serum as a means to treat diphtheria patients. In what is considered the first major therapeutic breakthrough of the bacteriological era, Behring and Kitasato demonstrated that nonlethal doses of diphtheria toxin induced mammals to form substances that would neutralize the activity of the injected toxin. These substances, or antitoxins, were protective antibodies, eventually leading to the concept of serum therapy and passive immunization against diphtheria (and other diseases) and the discovery of humoral immunity.

Behring and others, notably German scientist Paul Ehrlich, went on to produce antitoxin by inoculating horses with repeated injections of filtered toxin in order to harvest immune serum. As a result, diphtheria at last became treatable. In 1901 Behring was awarded the first Nobel Prize in Physiology or Medicine "for his work on serum therapy, especially its application against diphtheria."

Behring's antitoxin was first successfully marketed in 1892 and quickly became routine therapy. Collaboration with Ehrlich had been essential to understanding acquired immunity to disease in animals and contributed to making Behring's breakthrough discovery clinically applicable. Ehrlich had proposed the use of large animals such as horses for commercial production of diphtheria antiserum. More importantly, he developed a technique to standardize the potency of serum antitoxin with respect to antibody concentration. Quantifying immunity as the "multiple" of the lethal dose of a toxin tolerated by the immunized animal, he provided the basis for standardizing diphtheria antitoxin and producing it on an industrial scale. Ehrlich's work on antigens and

The Great Race of Mercy

In 1925, Nome physician Curtis Welch witnessed several young patients die of what he thought was severe tonsillitis. As cases multiplied and more children developed sore throats and respiratory distress, Welch saw the tell-tale gray pseudo-membrane of diphtheria. Nome and much of Northwest Alaska had been struck by an epidemic of diphtheria.

Welch had no fresh antitoxin supply. With the mayor of Nome he quarantined the town and put out an urgent call for diphtheria antitoxin. In winter, Nome, situated just below the Arctic Circle, was only accessible by the Iditarod Trail, 1,600 km traversing the vast dangerous interior of Alaska. The nearest batch of antitoxin was that far away in Anchorage. Nome's frozen harbor made sea transport impossible, and open-cockpit airplanes could not fly in Alaska's subzero temperatures. The only way to obtain a supply of the lifesaving medicine would be by dog sled; sleds regularly delivered mail over Alaska's snowbound territories. So Governor Bone recruited the best drivers and dog teams for a nonstop relay to transport the serum.

Anchorage Hospital agreed to ship its 300,000 units of antitoxin on hand by train to Nenana, over 1,000 km from Nome. From there, the medicine would be transported by dog sled. In the evening of January 27, musher "Wild Bill" Shannon picked up the 20 pound, fur-wrapped package from the Nenana train station. Twenty teams of mushers and about 150 sled dogs took part in the ensuing 1,085-km relay journey. They battled extreme arctic temperatures, gale-force winds, and often near-blizzard conditions. Four dogs died of exposure, and several mushers suffered severe frostbite.

The lifesaving antitoxin reached Nome on February 2. Five children had already died. But many others survived, and three weeks later the quarantine was lifted. The heroic feat of the mushers and their dog teams received national attention and became known as the *Great Race of Mercy*, or the *Nome Serum Run*.

The Serum Run helped spur the Kelly Act, signed into law in 1925, allowing private aviation companies to bid on mail delivery contracts. Within a decade, airmail routes were established in Alaska. The last U.S. Post Office dog sled route closed in 1963. Today, the popular Iditarod Trail Sled Dog Race has revitalized mushing as a sport and traditionally honors the participants in the historic Serum Run to Nome.

antibodies laid the foundation of modern immunology and earned him the Nobel Prize for Medicine in 1908.

In 1907, Behring showed that a mixture of diphtheria toxin and antitoxin produced immunity to diphtheria in humans. However, the combination of toxin-antitoxin needed to be carefully balanced so as to provide enough toxin to elicit active immunity, yet enough antitoxin to prevent disease. The main problem with this type of immunization was its short-term protective effect, lasting only a few months. It was useful during epidemics and to treat acute infections, but posed dosage risks and did not prevent disease. In order to avert these dangers, researchers were experimenting with other nontoxic forms of antitoxin to be used for safe and effective mass vaccination.

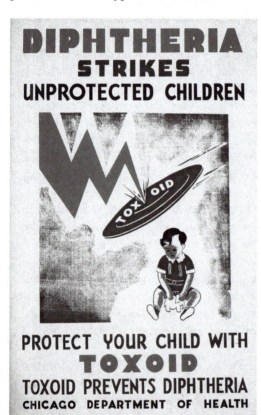

Public service advertisement, ca. 1936–1941. Diphtheria toxoid immunization became increasingly widespread starting in the 1930s. While the disease has not been eradicated, it is very rare in developed countries today. In 2015, Spain reported its first fatal case in three decades, in a six-year-old child. (Library of Congress)

In 1914, American physician William Park (1863–1939) succeeded in formulating a diphtheria toxin–antitoxin preparation that optimized lasting immunity while causing minimal adverse reactions. His mixture was used for immunization until the advent of diphtheria toxoid developed by Pasteur veterinarian Gaston Ramon in 1922. By treating diphtheria toxin with heat and formalin, Ramon successfully inactivated the toxin so that it could no longer destroy cells and cause disease, but still induce formation of antibodies that would block natural toxins.

Completely nontoxic, this substance had the same antigenic potency as the natural toxin and provided the simplest and most effective way to prevent diphtheria. First named anatoxin, it was eventually called diphtheria toxoid.

Vaccinations using formaldehyde-detoxified diphtheria toxoid began in 1924. Their efficacy was quickly confirmed and recommended immunization procedures established. Ramon's revolutionary substance was the first example of what became later known as "chemical" or "subunit" vaccines and ushered in the modern era of toxoid vaccines. Today, diphtheria vaccine (diphtheria toxoid) is still manufactured in many countries using Ramon's original procedure with only minor refinements. Ramon also pioneered the use of adjuvants to enhance immune response. In 1926, British physician Alexander Glenny found that use of aluminum potassium, or alum, delayed absorption from the site of injection and induced higher antibody production. Aluminum salts remain the most commonly used vaccine adjuvants in human vaccines.

Nowadays, diphtheria toxoid is widely used as a component of DPT (diphtheria, pertussis, tetanus) vaccine and is approximately 95 percent effective. Immunization with antigenically intact toxoid changed diphtheria from a dangerous, often fatal childhood disease into an extremely rare occurrence in the developed world. However, the bacillus has not been entirely eradicated. A 1990 outbreak, which occurred after the dismantling of the former Soviet Union, resulted in over 15,000 cases in the Russian Federation and nearly 3,000 in the Ukraine and demonstrated the persistence of diphtheria as a potential serious health hazard in settings of social unrest and inadequate healthcare infrastructure. Between 2000 and 2008, the World Health Organization reported several thousand annual cases, further evidence that microbial reservoirs still exist.

Penicillin, antitoxin, and maintaining an open airway are paramount in treating toxigenic diphtheria; even so, a small percentage of cases are fatal. Therefore, mass immunization is essential for disease control.

Bibliography and Suggested Readings

Burkovski, Andreas, "Diphtheria and Its Etiological Agents," in *Corynebacterium Diphtheriae and Related Toxigenic Species*, ed. Andreas Burkovski, Dordrecht: Springer Netherlands, 2014, pp. 1–14 and 225–238.

Carmichael, Ann G., "Diphtheria," in *Cambridge World History of Human Disease*, ed. Kenneth F. Kiple, Cambridge: Cambridge University Press, 1993, pp. 680–683.

Centers for Disease Control and Prevention, 2015, "The Pink Book: Diphtheria," http://www.cdc.gov/vaccines/pubs/pinkbook/dip.html.

Drews, Jürgen, "Paul Ehrlich: Magister Mundi," *Nature Reviews* September 2004, 3: 797–801.

Rappuoli, Rino, and Malito, Enrico, "History of Diphtheria Vaccine Development" in *Corynebacterium Diphtheriae and Related Toxigenic Species*, ed. Andreas Burkovski, Dordrecht: Springer Netherlands, 2014, pp. 1–14 and 225–238.

Insulin

What	*Synthetic version of* a hormone produced by the pancreas and essential for normal carbohydrate metabolism.
Where	Canada
When	1921–1922
By Whom	Frederick Banting (1891–1941); Charles Best (1899–1978); John MacLeod (1876–1936); James Collip (1892–1965)
Importance	Lifesaving treatment for diabetic patients who until then had been doomed to premature death; important contribution to the understanding of physiology of digestion; major advance in the field of endocrinology.

Scientists had recognized the nature of the pancreas as a digestive gland as early as the 17th century. German medical student Paul Langerhans in 1869 first described the distinct clusters of pancreatic cells now known as the insulin-producing *islets of Langerhans*. In the 1870s French pharmacist Apollinaire Bouchardat, recognized for his work on a diabetic diet and exercise regimen, had speculated that the source of diabetes was malfunction of the pancreas. The first experimental evidence connecting the pancreas and diabetes was uncovered in 1889 when Strasbourg scientists Oskar Minkowski and Joseph von Mering found that total pancreatectomy in dogs resulted in severe diabetes.

Subsequent experiments with animals of different species confirmed these findings: removal of the pancreas led to glycosuria and fatal wasting. The link of the pancreas to diabetes was thus established. Mering and Minkowski concluded that "diabetes, as observed after the total removal of the pancreas, can only be the result of a cessation of a function of this organ, which for the consumption of sugar in the organism is absolutely necessary. This means that we have to reckon with *a special, so far still unknown, function of the pancreas* [original emphasis]."

In 1901, the American pathologist Eugene Opie, while a student at Johns Hopkins, noted morbid changes in the pancreatic islet cells of diabetic patients. English physiologist Edward A. Sharpey-Schäefer, hypothesizing that the islets of Langerhans produced an *endocrine* secretion (one fed directly into the bloodstream) capable of regulating carbohydrate metabolism, in 1913 coined the word *insulin* (from the Latin *insula*, island) to name this as yet unidentified new substance.

Attempts to treat diabetes began as soon as the role of the pancreas in glucose metabolism was recognized. Many researchers tried to give pancreatic extract to animal and human diabetics, but most of these early experiments resulted in failed or even harmful outcomes. Pancreatic extracts were difficult to purify, and although they could lower blood sugar and reduce glycosuria, toxic reactions prevented their use in humans. Georg Zuelzer in Germany, E. L. Scott and Israel Kleiner in the United States, and Nicolas Paulescu in Romania were among those who broke new ground. Both Kleiner and Paulescu independently demonstrated that intravenous injection of their extract, a solution of fresh pancreas in lightly salted distilled water, led to dramatic decreases in blood and urinary sugar and ketones. Their work was interrupted by the outbreak of World War I. Kleiner left the Rockefeller Institute and did not continue his attempts to isolate the "antidiabetic factor." Paulescu had come close to purifying insulin, but Austrian occupation and the turmoil of the early postwar era in Bucharest delayed his work for several years.

In the end, the active principle secreted by the islet cells was successfully isolated in John MacLeod's physiology laboratory at the University of Toronto by young Ontario surgeon Frederick Banting and his assistant Charles Best. Banting had been given laboratory space by MacLeod to investigate the function of the pancreatic islets. He was to test his hypothesis that ligation of the pancreatic ducts *in vivo* would destroy the enzyme-secreting parts of the organ, but leave intact the islets of Langerhans believed to produce the substance regulating sugar metabolism. Charles Best and Clark Noble were the two student assistants MacLeod had assigned to work with Banting over the summer. Best and Noble flipped a coin to see who would work with Banting first; Best won the coin toss.

During the summer of 1921, Banting and his student performed a series of experiments combining pancreatic duct ligation with the complete surgical removal of the pancreas. After weeks of laborious setbacks, Banting's idea, namely the extraction and isolation of such secretions as were produced after degeneration of the acinar cells in duct-ligated animals, finally bore fruit. In the fall of 1921, the team reported that they were keeping a moribund diabetic dog alive with injections of pancreatic extract, prepared in a saline solution according to MacLeod's instructions. The extract, which they had named "isletin," dramatically lowered the blood sugar levels of their experimental dogs.

On December 30, 1921, Macleod, Banting, and Best first presented their findings at the conference of the American Physiological Society in New Haven, Connecticut. Around the same time, biochemist James Collip was invited to join the team to help purify their pancreatic extract for clinical testing in human patients.

In January 1922 Collip's purified extract was injected into Leonard Thompson, a 14-year-old Toronto boy who was dying of diabetes. The injections produced remarkable and rapid improvement. Within days, the boy's blood sugar dropped dramatically and his glucose excretion decreased nearly 10-fold. He looked and felt better and became more active. This was the first clearly successful test of the new substance on a human diabetic.

The following month six more patients were treated, all with favorable outcomes. A subsequent series of clinical studies defined the biological effects of insulin and established guidelines for its clinical use. The success of these clinical results was such as to leave no doubt in Banting's mind that the extracts provided "a therapeutic measure of unquestionable value in the treatment of certain phases of the disease in man."

Banting and MacLeod were awarded the 1923 Nobel Prize in Physiology or Medicine "for the discovery of insulin"; they shared their prize with Best and Collip. The Nobel Committee had concluded that the discovery was Banting's idea alone, but that "it was Macleod's guiding hand that helped Banting's idea reach such a happy culmination . . ." For the first time, as had been stipulated in Nobel's will, the award was given for a benefit conferred to mankind "during the preceding year."

The isolation of insulin at the University of Toronto in the winter of 1921–1922 was considered nothing short of miraculous. Before the discovery of insulin, the outlook for diabetic patients had been bleak. For centuries, the disease had been known as "the pissing evile, a melting down of the flesh into urine." The only treatment available was a starvation diet. At the turn of the 19th century, the average life expectancy for newly diagnosed diabetics ranged from one to eight years. These patients suffered from lowered resistance to infections, poor wound healing, early kidney failure, compromised eyesight, impaired circulation, and impotence. Now, even though there was as yet no cure for diabetes, the advent of insulin provided disease sufferers with an effective treatment and a new lease on life.

Bibliography and Suggested Readings

Banting, Frederick G., Best, Charles H., et al., "Pancreatic Extracts in the Treatment of Diabetes Mellitus," *Canadian Medical Association Journal* March 1922, 12(3): 141–146.

Bliss, Michael, *The Discovery of Insulin*, Chicago: University of Chicago Press, 1984.

Bliss, Michael, *The Making of Modern Medicine: Turning Points in the Treatment of Disease*, Chicago: University of Chicago Press, 2011.

Rosenfeld, Louis, "Insulin: Discovery and Controversy," *Clinical Chemistry* December 2002, 48(12): 2270–2288.

Sharpey-Schäfer, Edward. A., *An Introduction to the Study of the Endocrine Glands and Internal Secretions: Lane Medical Lectures, 1913, by Sir Edward Schäfer*, Stanford University: The University, 1914.

Von Mering, Joseph, and Minkowski, Oskar, "Diabetes mellitus nach Pankreasextirpation," *Centralblatt für klinische Medicin*, 1889, 10(23): 393–394.

Modern Psychopharmacology

What	The study and use of medications acting on specific neurotransmitters in order to treat psychiatric illnesses.
Where	France; Switzerland; United States
When	1950s and 1960s
By Whom	Jean Delay (1907–1987); Pierre Deniker (1917–1998); Nathan Kline (1916–1983); many others
Importance	Led to effective antipsychotic and antidepressant drugs; dramatically changed the practice of clinical psychiatry.

Modern psychopharmacology as a field of study dates from the introduction of the powerful antipsychotic chlorpromazine in 1952. Earlier, drugs such as chloral hydrate, bromides, and barbiturates, all developed in the 19th century, were used for the treatment of anxiety and insomnia and to sedate the mentally ill, but until the 1950s there was little innovation in clinical psychopharmacology. At the time, most practitioners did not endorse drug treatment of psychiatric problems but favored verbal psychotherapeutic interventions to improve patient functioning. It was not until the mid-20th century that advances in neuroscience, together with a growing pharmaceutical industry, began to fuel a biochemical approach in psychiatry.

The term "psychopharmacology," first coined at Johns Hopkins University in 1920, came into use at a time when psychoanalytic ideas and Freudian theories of disease causation had grown increasingly dominant in the treatment of psychiatric disorders. The 1952 discovery of the antipsychotic effects of chlorpromazine marked a turning point. Chlorpromazine, sold as Thorazine in the United States and elsewhere as Largactil, relieved the florid symptoms of severe schizophrenia—agitation, delusions, and hallucinations—and showed they could be controlled chemically. Moreover, chlorpromazine was not overly sedating, so for many patients it helped restore a measure of normal function.

Chlorpromazine is part of the phenothiazine family of compounds, first developed in 1880 and used as insecticides in the 1930s. In 1945, the French pharmaceutical company Rhône-Poulenc began studying a phenothiazine compound as a possible antihistamine. This resulted in the formulation of promethazine, still widely available today as Phenergan. One of its main side effects was marked sleepiness, indicating that it had central nervous system activity. French military surgeon Henri Laborit therefore began using promethazine to depress the autonomic nervous system to potentiate anesthesia and prevent shock. A related compound, chlorpromazine, was found to have both sedative and antipsychotic action.

Laborit's findings were confirmed serendipitously by psychiatrists Jean Delay and Pierre Deniker at Sainte-Anne Hospital in Paris, when their sedation therapy—a physical treatment consisting of lowering the body temperature with ice together with administering chlorpromazine—was suddenly disrupted because of ice shortage at the hospital. Delay and Deniker went on to conduct the first systematic clinical trials with the drug and quickly demonstrated its effectiveness in managing psychotic symptoms. They reported their findings in 1952, coining the term "neuroleptics" to designate an independent class of antipsychotic medications. Three years later, they convened the first international psychopharmacology meeting in Paris to discuss the new drug class.

Chlorpromazine was introduced in the United States as Thorazine in 1954. Thorazine was soon tried for multiple conditions, including pain, depression, anxiety, nausea, hyperactivity, and menopausal symptoms, although by 1970 the U.S. Food and Drug Administration limited its indications to psychosis. The drug was eventually adopted worldwide. It led to radical changes in many psychiatric hospitals where its effects on patients allowed initiation of social and even psychological therapies.

The clinical success of chlorpromazine ushered in a wave of other phenothiazine antipsychotics, paving the way for new explanations of psychosis and transforming psychiatric practice. Earlier so-called "physical" and often experimental or dangerous treatment methods such as insulin coma, shock and convulsive therapies, or even psychosurgery such as frontal lobotomy were largely abandoned and replaced with the prescription of psychotropic medications. By predictably relieving the "positive" symptoms of schizophrenia—disorganized thoughts and behaviors—the phenothiazines demonstrated that major mental illnesses were amenable to chemotherapy and that therefore such disorders must have a biological, chemically mediated basis in the brain. This was of great importance for the establishment of psychiatry as a medical science based on rational therapies rather than empirical approaches to syndromes.

Chlorpromazine appeared to work by blocking dopamine receptors in the brain, a discovery that led to the development of multiple antipsychotics with the same mechanism of action. Many had fewer antihistaminic and anticholinergic side effects and were also helpful in treating some of the "negative" symptoms of schizophrenia such as apathy or flat affect.

A further advance was the development in the late 1960s of long-acting injectable formulations. This made possible treatment of schizophrenic patients outside of hospital settings by eliminating the need for daily, closely supervised oral administration of medication. Together with reducing florid psychotic symptoms, long-acting injectable phenothiazines laid the practical foundation for what was to become the community mental health movement and the dismantling of state hospital systems. Hence the 1970s saw large numbers of psychiatric patients discharged from institutions into communities often ill prepared for the treatment and monitoring of the chronic mentally ill.

The early 1950s also witnessed the introduction of the first important family of agents effective in treating depression and anxiety. During a clinical trial of the antitubercular drug iproniazid, researchers had noted that some patients experienced "mild euphoria" and increased psychic energy. In fact, iproniazid inhibited monoamine oxidase, an enzyme that breaks down monoamines in the brain and thus extends bioavailability of these substances. It was yet another discovery that confirmed that neurotransmitters affected psychiatric disease. In 1957, U.S. psychiatrist Nathan Kline introduced the drug for the treatment of depressed patients. Iproniazid was ultimately found to be too toxic for clinical use, but other monoamine oxidase inhibitors (MAOIs) soon followed, notably phenelzine (Nardil) and tranylcypromine (Parnate). Clinical trials in the early 1960s established their effectiveness in depression and anxiety disorders.

In 1957 Swiss psychiatrist Roland Kuhn published the results of his observations on another new compound. This drug, imipramine, had no antipsychotic effects but resulted in remarkable improvement in patients with major depression. Canadian researcher Heinz Lehmann subsequently introduced imipramine to

North American psychiatry. Psychometric tests, together with a number of clinical studies, clearly showed the drug's efficacy and in 1959, imipramine, referred to as a tricyclic antidepressant because of its chemical structure, was successfully marketed as Tofranil. It was the first of a number of tricyclics to be launched and remains the gold standard of antidepressant therapy. In 1968, Swedish pharmacologist and later Nobel laureate Arvid Carlsson discovered that imipramine blocked nerve cell reuptake of the neurotransmitter serotonin.

These advances provided the impetus for further research into psychoactive medications. In 1960, chemist Leo Sternbach at Hoffmann La Roche in New Jersey developed chlordiazepoxide (Librium), the first of a highly effective class of antianxiety drugs known as benzodiazepines. Three years later the company launched diazepam, which was to become one of the most successful medications in prescription drug history. Marketed as Valium, it accounted for hundreds of millions of dollars in sales in the United States alone. A 1965 Rolling Stones's song enshrined the "little yellow pill" in popular culture as *Mother's Little Helper*.

Both Valium and Librium were useful in treating anxiety, phobias, and related conditions, as well as seizure and withdrawal syndromes, and by the end of the 20th century dozens of derivative compounds were marketed worldwide. Benzodiazepines have been among the most effective agents in the history of psychopharmacology. They are relatively safe and remain the anxiolytic of choice, even though today they are often avoided because of their potential addictiveness.

In the 1990s the study of serotonin led to the marketing of another class of drugs, based on the theory that inhibiting serotonin "reuptake" in the brain, at the synaptic junction between neurons, might bring relief in depression and other states, especially obsessive-compulsive disorder (OCD). By inhibiting reabsorption, these drugs, known as selective serotonin reuptake inhibitors, or SSRIs, would increase the amount of serotonin available at the synapse and thus relieve psychiatric symptoms. The first SSRI had been patented in 1972 as zimelidine. Further SSRIs followed, of which the most successful was fluoxetine. Initially intended for weight loss and patented in 1975, it was launched for depression in 1988 under the brand name Prozac; it would become one of the most successful psychopharmacological products of the era.

The introduction in the 1950s and 1960s of the first truly effective medications to treat psychosis and mood disorders has transformed psychiatry. The success of such drugs as chlorpromazine, imipramine, and the benzodiazepines increasingly oriented clinical psychiatry toward pharmaceuticals rather than psychotherapy. At the same time, understanding the mechanism of action of psychotropic drugs has become essential and requires advanced knowledge of central neurotransmitters, their metabolism, and their psychophysiological significance. Drugs that block dopamine transmission are therapeutic in psychotic states such as schizophrenia; depression, on the other hand, attributed to a deficiency of neuronal monoamines—dopamine, norepinephrine, and serotonin—is alleviated by raising their levels.

A growing body of biochemical knowledge derived from the use of psychiatric drugs is therefore at the basis of modern theories of mental illness. These theories have largely come to rest on psychopharmacology itself and on understanding how pharmaceuticals that treat mental symptoms affect brain chemistry.

Bibliography and Suggested Readings

Healy, David, *Creation of Psychopharmacology*, Cambridge: Harvard University Press, 2002.

Jean-Gaël, Barbara, "History of Psychopharmacology: From Functional Restitution to Functional Enhancement," in *Handbook of Neuroethics*, eds. Jens Clausen and Neil Levy, Dordrecht: Springer Netherlands, 2015.

Shorter, Edward, *Historical Dictionary of Psychiatry*, Cary: Oxford University Press, 2005.

Shorter, Edward, *Before Prozac: The Troubled History of Mood Disorders in Psychiatry*, Cary: Oxford University Press, 2008.

Penicillin

What	Antibiotic drug derived from a mold of the genus *Penicillium*. Part of the beta-lactam group of antibiotics, penicillin works by inhibiting synthesis of the bacterial cell wall, thus preventing bacterial growth and division and ultimately causing cell death.
Where	England
When	1928
By Whom	Alexander Fleming (1881–1955); Howard Florey (1898–1968); Ernst Boris Chain (1906–1979)
Importance	First drug to be effective in treating a number of severe infectious diseases, including dangerous staphylococcal and streptococcal infections, gonorrhea, and syphilis.

The discovery of penicillin marked a major turning point in medical history. A natural substance derived from molds of the *Penicillium* family, and one of the earliest modern antibiotics, it proved to be a powerful drug that enabled doctors to treat previously incurable infections.

In ancient medicine, molds and fungi had long been credited with therapeutic activity. Traditional remedies made from plants, soil, and molds were used to treat certain conditions, especially superficial infections and skin conditions. In ancient China, as in Egypt and Greece, moldy bread crusts were applied to dress deep wounds or cuts. Retrospectively, these empiric therapies may have "worked" because of a basic antibiotic action of the bread mold.

In 1877, Louis Pasteur, having observed growth patterns of anthrax bacilli in nonsterile media, introduced the notion that biological agents might serve to destroy disease-causing bacteria. His concept of bacterial antagonism, namely that one infectious agent could inhibit or kill another, was later termed "antibiosis" by the French mycologist Paul Vuillemin. American biochemist and microbiologist Selman Waksman was the one who ultimately coined the word "antibiotic" (from the Greek, "against life") to describe substances that would be antagonistic to the growth of microorganisms.

The antimicrobial action of penicillin first came to light in 1928 through the work of Scottish bacteriologist Alexander Fleming. Three decades earlier Ernest Duchesne, a French medical student, had noticed the therapeutic properties of molds while working at the Lyon Military Hospital. There, stable boys used mold to help heal their horses' saddle sores. Duchesne conducted a series of experiments on the antagonism between molds and microbes and found that injecting a mold solution protected an animal infected with typhoid bacilli. The scientific community largely ignored the young man's 1897 doctoral thesis on the topic. Unfortunately, army service prevented Duchesne's continued research, and in 1912 he died prematurely of presumed tuberculosis.

In 1928, Alexander Fleming, a biologist at St. Mary's Hospital in London, had been investigating *Staphylococcus aureus*, a microbe commonly responsible for abscesses, when he discovered upon returning from holiday that an unattended plate culture had been contaminated by a mold. Upon closer examination, it appeared that the colonies of staphylococci adjacent to the mold had been destroyed. To confirm this, Fleming started growing the mold in pure culture. He found that it indeed produced a substance capable of inhibiting bacterial growth, including that of pathogenic gram-positive organisms (named after the special staining method developed by bacteriologist J. M. Gram), such as staphylococci, streptococci, and meningococci. These were and still are the deadly agents responsible for bacterial pneumonia, meningitis, and many wound infections.

Fleming also found that this unknown substance had no toxic effect on healthy tissue and did not interfere with white blood cell function, essential in defense against infection. He eventually named it *penicillin* and in 1929 published the results of his studies in the *British Journal of Experimental Pathology*. There he noted that his "mould broth" might have therapeutic value if the active substance—penicillin—could be isolated and produced. However, penicillin proved unstable and difficult to make, and therefore seemed to hold little clinical promise.

There was virtually no further research until 1938, when Oxford scientists Howard Florey, Ernst Boris Chain, and Norman Heatley undertook a project on antibacterial substances and came across Fleming's study. They started culturing Fleming's mold, *Penicillium notatum,* and were able to isolate enough of the active penicillin ingredient to test its efficacy in mice. Of the mice they inoculated with lethal streptococci, all who were treated with penicillin survived, thus demonstrating the antibacterial properties and therapeutic potential of their substance. They next tried penicillin on a patient who was dying from staphylococcal septicemia. By the fourth day of therapy, the patient had greatly improved, but then their limited supply of penicillin ran out and the patient died.

Production difficulties persisted, in part due to limited resources of the British government during the early years of World War II. Unable to make sufficient quantities of penicillin in their laboratory, Florey and Heatley turned to the United States for help. In 1941 they transferred their work to the North Regional Research Laboratory in Peoria, Illinois, where various fermentation methods to increase growth rates of fungal cultures were being investigated. Soon, using large beer vats for their experiments, Heatley and Andrew Moyer, the laboratory expert on fungal nutrition, were able to increase the yield of their penicillin cultures more than 30-fold.

The benefits of the new drug quickly became manifest. In Britain in 1942, Howard Florey's wife Ethel supervised systematic experiments conducted on airmen recovering from severe burns and on patients with infections of the eye and of the mastoid bone. In the United States the same year, penicillin was used for the first time on large numbers of civilians in the aftermath of the Cocoanut Grove disaster, a horrific fire at a Boston supper club that claimed nearly 500 victims. Many of the badly burned survivors were saved.

By 1943, the effectiveness of the new anti-infectious agent was unquestioned. That year, Howard Florey had traveled to North Africa to test penicillin on war wounds and was able to prevent infection by putting penicillin powder into a wound. Penicillin in 1943 also reportedly saved the life of actress Marlene Dietrich; she had contracted pneumonia while entertaining Allied troops in

Bari, Italy. Similar dramatic findings in the United States convinced both American and British pharmaceutical companies to expand their production of penicillin.

The urgent need for medicines to combat infections in the Allied forces drove unprecedented industrial collaboration on both sides of the Atlantic. Ramped-up mass production allowed widespread distribution of penicillin to the military and the general public. By D-Day in June 1944, enough was available to provide for the treatment of many Allied soldiers. At the same time, advances in product purification and medicinal formulation were made possible by increased scientific understanding of the chemical nature of the drug.

Penicillin proved to be highly effective against many previously intractable conditions: purulent infections caused by staphylococci; bacterial pneumonia and meningitis; and diphtheria, anthrax, tetanus, and rheumatic fever, the bane of childhood streptococcal infection. It was also very successful in treating gonorrhea and syphilis, two sexually transmitted infections that had always been major threats in times of war, when young men were far from home and at greater risk of being infected. In 1943, the director of the venereal disease research lab at New York's Marine Hospital had tested penicillin on four Navy men infected with syphilis with spectacular results. This gave further impetus to U.S. mass production, leading a project director to note that the goal was "to make penicillin so cheaply that it costs less to cure [syphilis] than to get it!"

As a result of their work in the development of penicillin as a therapeutic agent, Fleming, Florey, and Chain were awarded the 1945 Nobel Prize. Andrew Moyer, in 1948, was granted a patent for his method of the mass production of penicillin. Norman Heatley was recognized in 1990 with the first honorary MD ever given in the history of Oxford University.

Bibliography and Suggested Readings

Bud, Robert, *Penicillin: Triumph and Tragedy*, Oxford: Oxford University Press, 2007.

Fleming, Alexander, "On the Antibacterial Action of Cultures of a *Penicillium,* with Special Reference to Their Use in the Isolation of *B. influenza*," *British Journal of Experimental Pathology* 1929, 10: 226–236.

Hatfield, Gabrielle, *Encyclopedia of Folk Medicine: Old World and New World Traditions*, Santa Barbara: ABC-CLIO, 2004.

Markel, Howard, "The Real Story Behind Penicillin," 2013, http://www.pbs.org/new shour/rundown/2013/09/the-real-story-behind-the-worlds-first-antibiotic.html.

Porter, Roy, *The Greatest Benefit to Mankind*, London: Harper Collins, 1997.

Sykes, Richard, "Penicillin: From Discovery to Product," *Bulletin of the World Health Organization* 2001, 8: 78–79.

Polio Vaccine

What	Biological substance providing active acquired immunity against poliomyelitis.
Where	United States
When	1953; 1955
By Whom	Hilary Koprowski (1916–2013); Jonas Salk (1914–1995); Albert Sabin (1906–1993)
Importance	Medical advance that addressed a major public health problem and made possible near-eradication of polio throughout the world.

Poliomyelitis, also known as infantile paralysis, is a highly contagious viral infection, leading to inflammation and destruction of motor neurons. The virus multiplies in the gastrointestinal tract and is most often transmitted through fecal-oral contact, but also spreads through oral or nasal secretions of an infected person. Its effects range from mild to severe and may lead to permanent disability and death. The disease had existed for thousands of years but was virtually unknown before the 1900s when it became endemic in Europe and North America. For reasons that are unclear, it reached epidemic proportions in the early 20th century and by 1920, outbreaks had become regular events, primarily during the summer months. From the 1920s to the 1950s there were outbreaks of polio in various European countries, but it was in the United States that the disease struck most cruelly. In spite of stringent public health measures, a 1916 epidemic led to 27,000 cases nationwide, including 6,000 deaths with over 2,000 in New York City alone. In 1952, there were approximately 58,000 reported cases. Of those, according to U.S. Public Health Service records, 3,145 died and 21,269 suffered paralysis.

Polio struck indiscriminately and could cripple or kill. When the disease invaded the central nervous system, it caused meningitis, weakness (paresis), or paralysis of one or more muscle groups, depending on the site of infection; if it affected the brainstem, which controls the muscles of respiration, death usually ensued. Young children were polio's primary victims. Mortality was about 5 percent. Of the survivors, some recovered use of their muscles in the months following acute infection, but most remained permanently disabled.

Fear of the disease gave rise to widespread panic among parents of young children. Parks and swimming pools were closed, crowds avoided, and children kept home from school; as in prior plagues, thousands of frightened city dwellers fled to nearby country resorts. The threat of sudden, unpredictable death or of permanent disability and lifelong dependency galvanized unprecedented public response in search for a cure. Public health administrators and physicians, applying earlier tenets of epidemic controls, blamed crowded urban conditions and poor hygiene for the spread of the disease and imposed a variety of quarantine measures. Paradoxically, modern science has attributed the rise of polio to improved living conditions. Indeed, it is now thought that infants and children who in earlier, less "hygienic," eras were exposed to the virus at a young age, developed mild, subclinical infections that were protective. Subsequent generations growing up without this protective early exposure were at greater risk and often suffered the paralytic form of polio.

When Franklin Delano Roosevelt, future governor of New York and president of the United States, contracted paralytic polio in 1921, efforts to fight the

A Pennsylvania Boy Remembers the Polio Years

"Growing up before the anti-Polio shots could be scary. At school, someone always seemed to be in some sort of brace, or limping around, dragging a leg. The ones who made a good recovery frequently became stars on the swim team because of all the PT they had had, which led into swimming competitively; even so, many still limped while walking. Worse yet, some kids got sick and never came back to school.

Summer was a challenge. Parents were frightened by swimming pools, and the ones that were open were hyper-chlorinated. Larger bodies of water were considered safer but probably were not. Somehow the contagion was associated with elimination. Pools usually required showering before entering. At a private boys' school summer camp, the pool director insisted on kids swimming in the nude, and routinely inspected their rumps before allowing them to jump in!

Fundraising for polio research was everywhere, spearheaded by the March of Dimes. Local hospitals held raffles to fund the purchase of iron lungs, great glass and metal tubes into which kids who couldn't breathe were placed. In fact, the apparatus looked really terrifying. So we pestered our parents to escape from contagion by 'going down the Jersey Shore.' Salt water seemed safer, or maybe it was the waves. When Dr. Salk's Vaccine hit "ole Doc's" office, no one cried . . . in fact we all ran down to get in line!"

Personal Statement by R. F., b. 1938. Used by permission.

disease gained national attention. They culminated in the establishment of the National Foundation for Infantile Paralysis (NFIP), which eventually brought massive funding to polio research. Promoted as the "March of Dimes," the compelling campaigns of the National Foundation not only publicized and popularized scientific advances, but also came to symbolize the power of countless small individual donations.

The agent of polio, first identified in 1908 by Karl Landsteiner and Erwin Popper, was not a bacterium, but a "filterable virus" small enough to pass through a porcelain filter. This discovery set the stage for future research. Soon, it was shown that the serum of monkeys artificially infected with polio contained "germicidal substances," namely antibodies. The same neutralizing substances were found in the blood of convalescent human patients, but it would

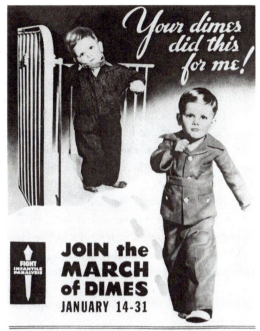

THE NATIONAL FOUNDATION FOR INFANTILE PARALYSIS, INC.
FRANKLIN D. ROOSEVELT, FOUNDER

Donald Anderson, born October 1, 1940, the first polio victim to be pictured on a 1946 March of Dimes publicity poster, giving rise to the popular phrase "poster child." He had contracted polio at the age of three, and was five years old at the time this iconic image came to symbolize the fight against polio. Founded in 1938 by Franklin D. Roosevelt as the National Foundation for Infantile Paralysis, the March of Dimes continues to promote maternal and child health. (AP Photo/ PRNewsFoto/March of Dimes)

take another four decades before a safe and reliable method of preventing the disease was developed.

In 1948, Harvard microbiologist John Enders and colleagues Frederick Robbins and Thomas Weller first succeeded in growing poliovirus in cultures of various types of tissue. Using cells derived not only from nervous tissue but from skin, muscle, and intestine, they showed that the virus was not a strictly neurotropic agent, that is, capable only of multiplying in nerve cells as had previously been thought. They also found that virus multiplication led to cell changes and destruction, which made it easier to interpret culture results. Immune serum inhibited viral growth, which made their technique applicable to immunity testing. Enders and his colleagues were awarded the 1954 Nobel Prize in Physiology or Medicine for their groundbreaking work.

Meanwhile, researchers had also discovered three distinct strains of the virus; for any vaccine to be effective, it would therefore have to provide immunity against all three. Enders's new technique of tissue cultivation was successful in cultivating all three strains outside the animal body, thus clearing the way for the development of a vaccine.

A dilute poliovirus vaccine had been tested as early as 1935, but several recipients developed polio and six of them died. In 1950, the NFIP, encouraged by the work of Enders and others including virologist Hilary Koprowski, renewed efforts to find a safe vaccine. In the late 1940s, Koprowski had developed a live oral polio vaccine by attenuating virus in rat brain cells. He had administered the preparation first to himself, then, in 1950, to 20 institutionalized disabled children; 17 developed antibodies to poliovirus and none developed complications.

In 1952 and 1953, National Foundation grantee Jonas Salk of the University of Pittsburgh reported successful preliminary testing of his killed, formalin-inactivated poliovirus preparation. The following year, the new Salk vaccine was tested on 1,830,000 experimental subjects and controls in what was effectively the largest mass experiment in the history of medicine. The results announced in April 1955 showed that the vaccine was safe and effective—a major breakthrough in the fight against polio. Salk, the man whose laboratory magic saved the lives of children, became a national hero overnight, and his discovery fueled an extraordinary outpouring of public support for medical research. Contemporary media coverage has documented the speed and enthusiasm with which large-scale inoculations got under way. The same year, the Poliomyelitis Vaccination Act paved the way for nationwide vaccination programs.

Even while the Salk vaccine was hugely successful, the majority of virologists favored live vaccine. Indeed, Salk's inactivated killed vaccine required not just one, but three injections at consecutive intervals to guard against all three types of virus. It also conferred only short-term immunity lasting from one to two years, thus necessitating a booster in order to afford lasting protection. Live attenuated vaccine, on the other hand, could be administered orally, which greatly simplified mass immunization. Importantly, it also provided long-term, if not lifelong, immunity, just as did the disease itself.

Both forms of the vaccine did pose potential safety concerns. With the Salk method, there was the risk of incompletely inactivated virus, whereas with live attenuated vaccine there was the danger of reversion to virulence. The now infamous "Cutter Incident" confirmed these fears. In this instance, one of the worst pharmaceutical disasters in U.S. history, several lots of Salk vaccine manufactured by Cutter Laboratories in California contained active, virulent poliovirus in what were supposed to be batches of inactivated virus. Of the several thousand children inoculated with the vaccine and their contacts, nearly 200 developed paralytic polio and 10 died.

The live, attenuated virus vaccine eventually superseded the Salk vaccine. Albert Sabin at the University of Cincinnati had worked on developing his own preparation from one of Koprowski's strains. His proved to be the more attenuated, and thus less risky, and came into widespread use. Between 1955 and 1961, while waiting for approval of clinical trials in the United States, Sabin's oral vaccine was successfully tested on more than 100 million people in the Soviet Union and Eastern Europe, as well as in Singapore, Mexico, and the Netherlands. In 1958, the Soviet Union organized industrial production of oral poliovirus vaccine from Sabin strains and effectively became the first country to produce and broadly distribute this vaccine. As a result, poliomyelitis not only disappeared from the USSR within the first few years of its use, but also in Eastern Europe and Japan.

These successes abroad led to the initiation of clinical trials on 180,000 Cincinnati school children in 1960 and the subsequent U.S. licensing in 1961. Ultimately, in spite of considerable opposition from the March of Dimes Foundation, which had supported the Salk vaccine, the U.S. Public Health Service licensed Sabin's vaccine. Until then, the USSR and many other countries reaped the benefit of the Sabin vaccine, which although developed and financed by the United States, was not available there until 1961.

Together, the Sabin and Salk vaccines had dramatic results. They arrested polio epidemics in developed countries. Within the first few years, the incidence of paralytic polio fell more than 20-fold, from 14 per 100,000 in 1954 to 0.5 in 1961. Global efforts to eradicate polio initiated in 1988 by the World Health Organization have relied largely on the Sabin oral polio vaccine. By 1994, the disease was eradicated in the Americas, by 2000 in China and Australia, and in Europe by 2002. In 2015, polio remains endemic only in Nigeria, Afghanistan, and Pakistan; globally, the annual incidence today is approximately

2,000 cases. In the United States in 1990, polio survivors were estimated at 1.6 million.

The development of effective vaccines to prevent paralytic polio was one of the major medical breakthroughs of the 20th century. The legacy of poliomyelitis has persisted in expanded rehabilitation therapies, as well as in increased disability rights. The need to address functional deficits in survivors of paralytic polio also contributed to the development of many other technologies, from the early "iron lung" respirators to modern mechanical ventilation and other life-support measures, to reconstructive orthopedics, and rehabilitative physiotherapies and prosthetics.

Bibliography and Suggested Readings

Daniel, Thomas M., and Robbins, Frederick C., eds., *Polio*, Rochester: University of Rochester Press, 1997.

Gould, Tony, *A Summer Plague: Polio and Its Survivors, New Haven:* Yale University Press, 1995.

Hansen, Bert, *Picturing Medical Progress from Pasteur to Polio*, New Brunswick: Rutgers University Press, 2009.

Rogers, Naomi, *Dirt and Disease: Polio before FDR*, New Brunswick: Rutgers University Press, 1992.

World Health Organization, "Poliomyelitis (Polio)," http://www.who.int/topics/poliomyelitis/en.

Wyatt, Harold V., "Poliomyelitis," in *The Cambridge World History of Human Disease*, ed. Kenneth F. Kiple, Cambridge: Cambridge University Press, 1993, pp. 942–950.

Streptomycin

What	Antibiotic drug derived from a group of common soil bacteria called *actinomycetes*. Produced by the organism *Streptomyces griseus*, streptomycin is a bacteriocidal agent that inhibits the synthesis of vital proteins in both gram-positive and gram-negative microbes.
Where	United States
When	1943
By Whom	Albert Schatz (1920–2005); Selman Waksman (1888–1973)
Importance	First effective treatment for tuberculosis and a number of serious gram-negative infections; has helped save millions of lives.

Streptomycin, an antibiotic purified from the bacterium *Streptomyces griseus*, was first isolated in 1943 in the laboratory of soil microbiologist and biochemist Selman Waksman at Rutgers University. Selman Waksman had emigrated from his native Ukraine to the United States, where he obtained his PhD in biochemistry in 1918. At Rutgers, he studied soil protozoa and bacteria and became well known as a physiological soil microbiologist. When he heard of the effectiveness of penicillin, he changed the direction of his research from the study of soil fertility to that of actinomycetes, a group of soil bacteria, in the quest for antibiotics.

Waksman is said to have coined the term "antibiotic," and his lab ultimately discovered several antibiotic agents derived from actinomycetes. The first, actinomycin, was developed in 1940; streptomycin was discovered in 1943; neomycin and candicidin followed in 1949 and 1953. Streptomycin and neomycin found wide application in the treatment of a number of infectious diseases; neomycin is still used as a common topical antibacterial. Of the two, however, streptomycin would prove to be the most important. The second major antibiotic to be discovered after penicillin, it was the first to have significant activity against the tubercle bacillus and to cure tuberculosis (TB), a highly contagious disease that every year infected and killed millions of people worldwide.

Selman Waksman has generally been credited with the discovery of streptomycin. In 1952 he was awarded the Nobel Prize for his work. But Albert Schatz, a PhD student of Waksman at Rutgers, played a crucial role in the discovery. Schatz was the one who isolated the crucial streptomycin-producing strain of actinomycetes and who labored to extract and test the new antibiotic. He described the results of his studies in his 1945 doctoral thesis after first publishing them, together with Waksman, in a 1944 paper entitled "Streptomycin: A Substance Exhibiting Antibiotic Activity Against Gram Positive and Gram Negative Bacteria." The new substance, unlike penicillin, was capable of killing a number of gram-negative pathogens and, importantly, *Mycobacterium tuberculosis,* the cause of TB.

The next step was to test the effectiveness of streptomycin *in vivo*, first on animals, then on human subjects. This task fell to two medical researchers at the Mayo Clinic in Rochester, Minnesota, Drs. William Feldman and Cornwin Hinshaw. Feldman and Hinshaw had been evaluating the antitubercular effects of a number of experimental drugs for over a decade when they first started working with the Rutgers team in 1944. By then, the pharmaceutical company Merck, with whom Waksman had an agreement regarding antibiotics patent rights, had set up production of large quantities of purified streptomycin for use in clinical trials.

Over the course of the following year, Feldman and Hinshaw tested the new drug on guinea pigs inoculated with virulent tubercle bacilli. They were able to demonstrate not only its relatively low toxicity, but also the "unquestionable ability of streptomycin to reverse the potentially lethal course of . . . tuberculosis in guinea pigs . . ." They then went on to try the drug in tuberculosis patients at the Mineral Springs Sanatorium in Canon Falls, Minnesota. Their first successful cure was that of a 21-year-old woman with pulmonary tuberculosis; by the fall of 1946 they had treated over 30 cases of different forms of the disease. Soon after their pioneering work, large-scale clinical trials carried out by the Trudeau Society and the U.S. Veterans Administration Hospital, as well as an extensive randomized British study, proved beyond a doubt the effectiveness of streptomycin in the treatment of tuberculosis.

Most early accounts of the streptomycin discovery were written, or swayed, by Waksman. He made little reference to Albert Schatz, whose role in the process remained largely ignored even though the U.S. Patent Office had legally recognized Schatz as streptomycin's co-discoverer. Although it was clear that Waksman's research program and his search for therapeutic agents in soil microorganisms had led to the discovery of this antibiotic, it was Schatz, keen to find a compound active against tuberculosis, who had succeeded in isolating and producing the active streptomycin strain.

Albert Schatz eventually received a share of the royalties from the drug, but not until he brought suit against his former mentor. Nevertheless, he was denied just recognition for his contribution. The majority of the scientific establishment sided with Waksman, regarding Schatz as ungrateful, a "mere cog in a great wheel in the study of antibiotics in [Waksman's] laboratory." Waksman made no mention of Schatz in his autobiography, *My Life with the Microbes*, and the Nobel Committee reportedly was unaware of Schatz's role as co-discoverer when they awarded the prize to Waksman alone.

Bibliography and Suggested Readings

Epstein, Samuel, *Miracles from Microbes: The Road to Streptomycin*, New Brunswick: Rutgers University Press, 1946.

Hinshaw, Cornwin H., and Feldman, William H., "Streptomycin in Treatment of Clinical Tuberculosis: A Preliminary Report," *Proceedings of the Staff Meetings of the Mayo Clinic* 1945, 20: 313–317.

Pringle, Peter, *Experiment Eleven: Deceit and Betrayal in the Discovery of the Cure for Tuberculosis,* London: Bloomsbury, 2012.

Schatz, Albert, "The True Story of the Discovery of Streptomycin," *Actinomycetes* 1993, 4(2): 27–39.

Schatz, Albert, Bugie, Elizabeth, and Waksman, Selman, "Streptomycin: A Substance Exhibiting Antibiotic Activity Against Gram-Positive and Gram-Negative Bacteria," *Proceedings of the Society for Experimental and Biological Medicine* 1944, 55: 66–69.

Wainwright, Milton, *Miracle Cure: The Story of Penicillin and the Golden Age of Antibiotics*, Oxford: Basil Blackwell, 1990.

Wainwright, Milton, "Streptomycin: Discovery and Resultant Controversy," *History and Philosophy of the Life Sciences* 1991, 13: 97–124.

Waksman, Selman A., *The Literature on Streptomycin, 1944–1948,* New Brunswick: Rutgers University Press, 1948.

Waksman, Selman A., *My Life with the Microbes,* New York: Simon and Schuster, 1954.

Sulfa Drugs

What	First modern antimicrobial.
Where	Germany
When	1932
By Whom	Gerhard Domagk (1895–1964)
Importance	Revolutionized the treatment of infectious diseases; gave strong impetus to pharmaceutical research and led to a series of new drugs derived from sulfonamides.

Sulfa drugs, or sulfonamides, were the first synthetic chemicals effective against bacterial disease. Developed in the 1930s, at a time when death from infections such as pneumonia and blood poisoning was common, sulfonamides were considered miracle drugs. They marked a turning point in the history of medicine and ushered in a new era of chemotherapy to treat bacterial infections.

The antibacterial activity of sulfonamides was first discovered in the laboratories of I. G. Farben, a large German industrial conglomerate and producer of chemicals and dyes, through the work of pathologist Gerhard Domagk. Domagk, then director of the company's Institute of Pathology and Bacteriology, was engaged in an extensive project designed to test industrial chemicals for potential medicinal use. His collaborators, chemists Fritz Mietzsch and Josef Klarer, had already synthesized a number of dyes in the search for compounds that had specific affinity for both fibers and for microbial cells; they were aiming to develop a substance that would either damage these cells directly or "attack the conditions of their existence." They had found that adding a sulfonamide radical to certain dyes improved their quality and color-fastness.

In 1932, Domagk undertook the investigation of "prontosil rubrum," a red sulfonamide-containing dye newly synthesized by Mietzsch and Klarer. He hypothesized that this dye might bind to bacterial proteins and thus inhibit bacterial action. In a now-famous experiment, he infected laboratory mice with a strain of hemolytic streptococci isolated from a patient with fatal streptococcal sepsis. Within 48 hours, all his infected untreated controls had died, whereas infected mice treated with prontosil for three to five days survived, which demonstrated a specific chemotherapeutic effect against streptococci and the potential value of the new molecule in treating such infections.

By 1935, there was enough accumulated experience to confirm the efficacy of prontosil against serious streptococcal infections in humans, notably childbed fever, erysipelas, meningitis, and scarlet fever. Domagk had even treated his own daughter with a dose of prontosil for a severe streptococcal illness; the child made a full recovery. In February 1935, when reports were available from clinicians who had tested the new drug on patients, Domagk published the results of his experiments. His work quickly attracted worldwide attention.

Soon afterward, scientists at the Pasteur Institute in Paris, including Daniel Bovet, Jacques and Thérèse Tréfouël, and Frédéric Nitti, began conducting experiments on the mode of action of prontosil, replicating Domagk's animal model and testing multiple derivative compounds. They determined that the part of the dye molecule responsible for antibacterial activity was its sulfonamide component, sulfanilamide. This was a critical finding, for it not only established the efficacy of sulfanilamide alone—a simpler substance and less expensive to produce—but also one not covered by I. G. Farben's patent on prontosil. Sulfanilamide was a familiar chemical and could therefore be freely manufactured. The Pasteur team's breakthrough discovery paved the way for pharmaceutical companies in Europe and the United States to develop sulfa drugs of their own.

Meanwhile, the new drug was also gaining recognition in England and in the United States. In 1935, the Therapeutic Trials Committee charged London physician Leonard Colebrook with studying prontosil and its sulfonamide constituent. Colebrook's clinical results in cases of advanced puerperal sepsis, reported in late 1936, were spectacular. His studies also confirmed the Pasteur Institute findings that the bacteriostatic power of sulfonamides alone was superior to that of the prontosil compound: indeed the simpler compound was a metabolic product of the chemical reduction of prontosil in the body, which explained prontosil's lack of *in vitro* activity.

In the United States, after hearing of Colebrook's work with prontosil, Eleanor Bliss and Perrin Long at Johns Hopkins University undertook their own animal trials. They successfully tried the new drug to treat erysipelas and streptococcal meningitis. Still, most American physicians and the public at large only learned of the drug in December 1936, when sulfonamides cured the president's son, Franklin Roosevelt, Jr., of a severe streptococcal infection. Thereafter the U.S. medical and research communities embraced the new medicine. *Time* magazine hailed it as "the medical discovery of the decade." By spring 1937 multiple clinical and experimental trials were underway, as was production of sulfanilamide and related chemicals by more than a dozen British and American pharmaceutical companies. It is estimated that over 5,000 sulfa compounds were synthesized in the ensuing years, but only a fraction of them were shown to have antibacterial properties. Among the most important were sulfapyridine against pneumonia, sulfathiazole for sepsis, and sulfadiazine for urinary and intestinal tract infections.

Sulfonamides saved many lives. By the start of World War II, U.S. production output was over 700,000 lbs. On the front, sulfa drugs were used to fight diseases such as dysentery and septicemia. American soldiers were issued first aid belt-packs that included sulfa powder and were taught to sprinkle the powder immediately on any open wound to prevent infection. Sulfa powder and tablets were also chief components of the combat medic kit. Toward the end of the war, however, their use diminished, in part due to the advent of the less toxic penicillin and to the development of resistance in various bacterial strains.

Sulfa drugs are bacteriostatic, not bactericidal, antibiotics. They inhibit bacterial growth and multiplication by interfering with bacterial folic acid synthesis, essential for synthesis of DNA and microbial survival. Today their indications are limited. Sulfa formulations continue to be used mainly for uncomplicated urinary tract infections and for the topical treatment of burns. They are also effective in combating opportunistic AIDS pneumonia. Derivative compounds are utilized in the treatment of diabetes, hypertension, gout, and leprosy.

In the late 1930s the scientific world quickly recognized the great lifesaving benefits of sulfonamides, and Domagk's work laid the foundation for an extraordinary and rapid expansion of infectious disease chemotherapy. In 1939 Gerhard Domagk was awarded the Nobel Prize in Physiology or Medicine for his discovery of the antibacterial effects of prontosil. Nazi prohibitions, however, forced him to decline the award; he ultimately received his diploma and medal in 1947.

Bibliography and Suggested Readings

Brock, Thomas E., and Domagk, Gerhard, "A Contribution to the Chemotherapy of Bacterial Infections," *Reviews of Infectious Diseases* 1986, 8(1): 163–166.

Original German publication by Domagk, G., "Ein Beitrag zur Chemotherapie der bakteriellen Infektionen," *Deutsche Medizinische Wochenschrift* February 15, 1935, 61: 250–253.

Chemical & Engineering News, "Prontosil," https://pubs.acs.org/cen/coverstory/83/8325/8325prontosil.html.

Lesch, John E., *The First Miracle Drugs: How the Sulfa Drugs Transformed Medicine*, Oxford: Oxford University Press, 2007.

"Physiology or Medicine 1939—Presentation Speech," 2014, http://www.nobelprize.org/nobel_prizes/medicine/laureates/1939/press.html.

Other Important Discoveries

ABO Blood Groups

What	Major system of classification of human red blood cells (erythrocytes) based on inherited differences in specific surface antigens called A and B; all individuals have type A, B, O, or AB blood based upon the presence or absence of their red cell surface antigens.
Where	Austria
When	1901
By Whom	Karl Landsteiner (1868–1943)
Importance	Made possible safe therapeutic blood transfusions; advanced the fields of immunology and human genetics; paved the way for organ transplantation; and is used in medico-legal cases to resolve questions of disputed paternity.

Ever since it was discovered that blood circulates in a closed system within the body, scientists have experimented with the infusion into the bloodstream of various substances, including animal and human blood. It was quickly recognized that transfer of blood from one person to another for therapeutic purposes might be lifesaving, especially in cases of severe hemorrhage. Unfortunately, early transfusion attempts often led to fatal outcomes due to what is known today as an acute transfusion reaction caused by the breakdown, or hemolysis, of red blood cells.

In 1875 German physiologist Leonard Landois had observed agglutination and hemolysis during blood transfusion: when an animal was transfused with the blood of another animal species, the foreign blood cells clumped and broke up, releasing hemoglobin and other cell breakdown products into the circulation. In 1900, Austrian physician and immunologist Karl Landsteiner reported that similar reactions occurred when the blood of some people was mixed with that of others. He hypothesized that the agglutination, or clumping, of red blood cells that resulted from such an admixture was not a response to an infectious pathogen but might rather be due to an intrinsic incompatibility. He studied the blood of six laboratory colleagues and found that mixing serum and red cells of different individuals caused some samples to clump, whereas others did not. His results, published the following year, showed that the blood of healthy individuals could be categorized into specific groups on this basis. These observations led him to develop a system of three blood types, later named A, B, and C (eventually re-named O, for the German "*ohne*," without).

To explain the three groups, Landsteiner identified two antigens, A and B, and two antibodies, anti-A and anti-B: erythrocytes either had the A or B antigens, or fell into the O group, having neither A nor B. Group O blood, although devoid of A and B antigens, contained both anti-A and anti-B antibodies. In 1902, Landsteiner's colleagues Alfred von Decastello and Adriano Sturli described a fourth blood group, AB. In this group, both A and B antigens are present, whereas both anti-A and anti-B antibodies are absent.

Landsteiner's work received little attention until it became clear that transfusions between individuals of the same (homologous) blood groups did not result in the catastrophic transfusion reactions that often ensued. Indeed, jaundice, hemoglobinuria, shock, and fatal hemolysis only occurred when patients were transfused with heterologous blood, blood of a different type. In 1907, New York physician Reuben Ottenberg performed the first successful transfusion matching donor and recipient according to the ABO antigen system. Recognition of the ABO blood groups had made possible for the first time relatively safe and effective clinical transfusion procedures and had laid the foundation for transfusion medicine.

Scientific interest in Landsteiner's ABO system increased even more when Heidelberg scientists Ludwik Hirszfeld and Emil von Dungern in 1910 confirmed that blood group specificity was hereditary, as Landsteiner had suggested earlier. Indeed, blood types are handed down from parent to child in accordance with Mendelian laws. A and B antigenic specificities are inherited co-dominantly; both A and B antigens are dominant over O. This was the first proven example of the Mendelian inheritance of a normal human characteristic. It led to the use of ABO blood typing in medico-legal cases of disputed paternity, a significant advance in this field, even though the proof was of a negative character. Although blood-group determination cannot establish paternity, the principles governing dominant or recessive hereditary transmission can exclude it.

In 1940, Landsteiner, who had moved to the Rockefeller Institute for Medical Research, identified the Rh factor together with New York scientists Alexander Wiener and Philip Levine. This hereditary blood antigen, named for rhesus monkeys in which it was first discovered, is present in most humans.

Importantly, it was shown to be the cause of *erythroblastosis fetalis,* the much feared and previously not understood hemolytic disease of the newborn, which occurs when mother and fetus have Rh-incompatible blood types. The discovery led to initial treatment of babies with Rh disease with exchange transfusion. Now, this has been replaced by maternal prophylaxis with Rh immune globulin.

In 1930 Landsteiner was awarded the Nobel Prize in Physiology or Medicine for his discovery of human blood groups. Other blood groups were identified later, but the ABO blood group antigens, most immunogenic of all, remain of prime importance in transfusion medicine. ABO blood types are universally found throughout the world and are used for anthropological study of different populations. In spite of their clinical importance, however, the actual physiological function of the ABO blood group antigens remains unclear.

Bibliography and Suggested Readings

Dean, Laura, *Blood Groups and Red Cell Antigens*, Bethesda: National Center for Biotechnology Information, 2005.

Landsteiner, Karl, *The Specificity of Serological Reactions*, New York: Dover Publications, 1962.

"Physiology or Medicine 1930—Presentation Speech," http://www.nobelprize.org /nobel_prizes/medicine/laureates/1930/press.html.

Watkins, Winifred M., "The ABO Blood Group System: Historical Background," *Transfusion Medicine* August 2001, 11(4): 243–265.

Anesthesia

What	Insensitivity to pain (from the Greek, "without sensation"), a state achieved by administration of medicinal drugs before and during surgical operations.
Where	United States
When	1846
By Whom	William Thomas Green Morton (1819–1868); John Collins Warren (1778–1856)
Importance	Transformed surgery by making possible effective pain control and safe, complex operations; led to the development of the specialty of anesthesiology.

Until the advent of modern anesthesia, surgery had been limited by the lack of effective pain control. Doctors tried to dull pain with a variety of substances, including opiates, alcohol, and decoctions of hallucinogenic plants such as mandrake and henbane. Medieval records document surgical use of soporific sponges containing powdered opium and other hypnotics. However, none of these traditional analgesics and narcotics could safely induce sleep deep enough to permit thorough surgical exploration of internal organs or unhurried complex procedures. Constrained by patients' tolerance for pain, surgeons had to be quick rather than precise. Abdominal operations, including cesarean sections, were occasionally attempted, but most often the range of procedures was restricted to external or superficial conditions, amputations, or repair of fractures.

As anatomical and surgical science advanced, the need for safe pain control became even more pressing. By 1830, the early inhalants—ether, nitrous oxide, and chloroform—had been discovered but were not used for relief of pain. British chemist Humphry Davy, together with many others, had experimented with inhaling nitrous oxide, so-called "laughing gas," for social amusement; he noted that this seemed to relieve pain and might therefore be useful in surgical operations. In 1842, Georgia physician Crawford W. Long was reportedly the first to administer sulfuric ether, a volatile flammable liquid with properties similar to nitrous oxide, during three minor surgical procedures. In Connecticut, dentist Horace Wells learned of nitrous oxide in 1844 and inhaled it before having one of his own teeth removed; he subsequently built a special apparatus for its administration but was unable to demonstrate its usefulness.

In 1846, Boston dentist William Thomas Green Morton and surgeon John Collins Warren performed the first successful public trial of inhaled ether anesthesia in the surgical amphitheater of the Massachusetts General Hospital (now a National Historic Landmark and tourist attraction, known as the *Ether Dome*). Together they anesthetized a patient prior to removing a mass in his neck. News of their historic demonstration quickly spread to Europe where surgeons from Paris to Berlin adopted the new anesthetic. The same year, in a letter to Morton, American physician and writer Oliver Wendell Holmes coined the term "anesthesia" to describe the effect of ether inhalation.

Ether irritated the lungs, had a disagreeable odor, had a long induction period, and often caused nausea and vomiting. It was therefore soon abandoned for chloroform, first used in 1847 by Edinburgh surgeon James Young Simpson who discovered its narcotic properties during a lab accident. Chloroform, a colorless, sweet-smelling, and nonflammable volatile liquid, was more potent than ether and easier to use. Dripped onto a cloth or sponge held to the patient's nose, its inhalation produced rapid effects. John Snow attending Queen Victoria during the birth of her eighth child in 1853 famously administered the anesthetic to her with such success that the queen described the effect of "that blessed

Letter of Dr. Oliver Wendell Holmes to William T.G. Morton:

Boston, November 21, 1846
My Dear Sir:
Everybody wants to have a hand in a great discovery. All I will do is to give you a hint or two, as to names, or the name, to be applied to the state produced and the agent. The state should, I think, be called "anaesthesia." This signifies insensibility, more particularly (as used by Linnaeus and Cullen) to objects of touch. (See "Good-Nosology," p. 259.) The adjective will be "anaesthetic." Thus we might say the state of anaesthesia, or the anaesthetic state.

. . .

I would have a name pretty soon, and consult some accomplished scholar such as President Everett, or Dr. Bigelow, St., before fixing upon the terms, which will be repeated by the tongues of every civilized race of mankind.

. . .

You could mention these words, which I suggest for their consideration; but there may be others more appropriate and agreeable.

Yours respectfully,
O. W. Holmes.

Source: William C. Wile, *New England Medical Monthly, Volume 14.* Danbury: The Danbury Medical Printing Company, 1895, p. 202.

chloroform" as "soothing, quieting and delightful beyond measure." This regal *imprimatur* assured the acceptance of chloroform for use in childbirth despite widespread religious objections based on traditional biblical teaching that women should bring forth their children in pain. Chloroform was used on the battlefields of the Crimean War and the American Civil War, and for many years, until its cardiac and liver toxicities were fully appreciated, remained the anesthetic of choice.

In the 20th century, the search for more effective and safer inhalation anesthetics led to the use of fluorinated hydrocarbons, which were more stable, less flammable, and less toxic than ether or chloroform and their derivatives. Starting in 1951, halothane, then isoflurane, and finally, in 1992, desflurane were introduced. The latter, together with nitrous oxide, still remains a mainstay of inhalation anesthesia.

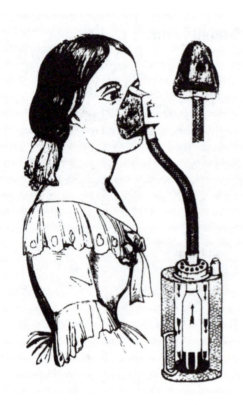

Nineteenth-century engraving of an early chloroform inhaler. Devised by English physician John Snow (who famously traced the 1853 London cholera epidemic to the Broad Street water pump), the apparatus had a dual-chamber cylinder connected by a flexible tube to a facemask, through which the patient inspired air charged with chloroform vapor. Snow discussed the dangers of simply giving the drug on a handkerchief in his 1848 book, *On Narcotism by the Inhalation of Vapours*. (De Agostini Picture Library/Getty Images)

So-called "open" administration of anesthetic agents via liquid droplets onto a gauze mask was replaced by closed, airtight systems, permitting better dosage control of the inhaled vapor. The introduction of endotracheal tubing prevented aspiration of secretions, and the addition of inflatable cuffs allowed positive pressure ventilation and regulation of the flow of oxygen and other gases into the lungs. Muscle relaxants further controlled respiratory movements. Low doses of the neuromuscular blocker curare (a plant alkaloid used as arrow poison in South America) produced profound flaccidity of striated muscle. First used successfully in Montreal in 1942, its rapidly reversible action made it an integral auxiliary to modern anesthesia, and especially useful for abdominal wall relaxation.

Not all operations required general anesthesia. Ethyl chloride spray produced a measure of localized numbing. Cocaine, the active ingredient of coca leaves first isolated in 1859, had anesthetic properties. Ophthalmologist Carl Koller in 1884 reported that the drug's topical application during eye operations rendered the cornea insensitive. The invention of the hollow needle some years earlier allowed for further development of regional anesthesia techniques. In the United States, surgeons William Halsted and Alfred Hall injected cocaine to achieve local anesthesia. In 1899 German surgeon August Bier performed the first spinal anesthesia, which was soon adopted for control of labor pains with fewer side effects. Bier also introduced a technique for regional intravenous anesthesia of the limbs, known as the Bier block. It involves the use of pneumatic tourniquets and is still used today in short operative procedures for the upper or lower extremities. In 1885 cocaine became the first local anesthetic to be synthesized by the Merck drug company, but its addictive nature led to its replacement with safer, less addicting agents such as procaine and lidocaine.

Intravenous anesthesia, first attempted in 1872 with chloral hydrate, gained increasing popularity. "Twilight sleep," a combination of intravenous morphine and scopolamine introduced during World War I, was abandoned due to serious side effects. The intravenous barbiturate thiopental, first used in 1932, proved to have significant cardiovascular depressant effects. Safer agents such as ketamine, etomidate, and propofol, introduced in 1977, eventually led to total intravenous anesthesia (TIVA). Importantly, the concept of "balanced anesthesia" introduced in the 1940s by Mayo Clinic physician John Lundy resulted in the use of low-dose combination regimens aiming to provide hypnosis, muscle relaxation, and analgesia while minimizing adverse side effects.

Over the course of the 20th century anesthesiology developed as a recognized medical specialty. Emphasis on intraoperative monitoring and safety in conjunction with effective pain control permitted surgeons to carry out increasingly complex and invasive procedures. Together with antiseptic techniques and asepsis, anesthesia revolutionized the field of surgery. Today, with pain no longer a barrier, surgery has become essential in modern patient care.

Bibliography and Suggested Readings

Gawande, Atul, "Two Hundred Years of Surgery," *New England Journal of Medicine* 2012, 366: 1716–1723.

Ortega, Rafael, and Mai, Christine, "History of Anesthesia," in *Essential Clinical Anesthesia*, eds. Charles Vacanti, Scott Segal, Pankaj Sikka, and Richard Urman, Cambridge: Cambridge University Press, 2011.

Pernick, Martin S., *The Calculus of Suffering: Pain, Professionalism, and Anesthesia in Nineteenth-Century America*, New York: Columbia University Press, 1985.

Porter, Roy, *The Greatest Benefit to Mankind: A Medical History of Humanity from Antiquity to the Present*, London: Harper-Collins, 1997.

Robinson, Daniel H., and Toledo, Alexander H., "Historical Development of Modern Anesthesia," *Journal of Investigative Surgery* 2012, 25: 141–149.

Antisepsis and Asepsis

What	Antimicrobial technique to destroy harmful microorganisms or inhibit their growth; from the Greek, "against putrefaction." Antiseptics are used to prevent infections of body tissues and to sterilize surgical instruments or other materials.
Where	Austria; England
When	1847; 1865
By Whom	Ignaz Semmelweis (1818–1865); Joseph Lister (1827–1912)
Importance	Revolutionized the practice of surgery and obstetrics; significantly reduced the incidence of surgical wound infections and postoperative morbidity and mortality; had a major impact on childbed fever and postpartum mortality.

The 19th-century discovery that some diseases were caused by living microscopic pathogens profoundly changed medical thought and practice. It took Pasteur to elucidate the exact nature of infectious disease, but the idea that sickness could be transmitted from person to person was ancient. We know that during medieval epidemics, public health strategies aimed to segregate and confine the sick. Clothing and personal belongings were sanitized with sulfur or altogether incinerated in order to ward off contagion. Anyone suspected of spreading disease was exiled or quarantined. As early as the 15th century, disease contagion was described as polluting "what it touches . . . and from the contact of one it reaches others very easily." Nevertheless, physicians long failed to grasp the link between observed person-to-person transmission and the systemic complications of wound infections or the deadly scourge of childbed fever.

Prior to surgical antisepsis, nearly half of all patients succumbed to wound infections. After giving birth, as many as one in five women were at risk of developing fatal postpartum sepsis. The 18th-century Scottish physician Alexander Gordon was among the first to recognize the infectious nature of childbed fever, but his findings were dismissed because they implied potential practitioner negligence. In 1843 Boston physician Oliver Wendell Holmes affirmed Gordon's observations, stating unambiguously that puerperal fever was *"so far contagious as to be frequently carried from patient to patient by physicians and nurses."* It was Ignaz Semmelweis, a Hungarian obstetrician, who in 1847 instituted the first effective measures to reduce the incidence of childbed fever. Semmelweis had noted that on the obstetrical wards of the Vienna *Allgemeines Krankenhaus* where medical students trained, mortality rates were as high as 20 percent. This was far higher than on the ward where midwives received their instruction; here, the death rates were, at most, 3 percent, an astonishing difference. The clinical training of the midwives did not include cadaver dissection, whereas medical students and their teachers came to the maternity ward straight from the autopsy room. These observations led Semmelweis to conclude that the infection might be carried from the dissected bodies of sepsis victims and contaminate healthy mothers. His suspicion was confirmed by the death of a colleague and friend from a wound infection he had sustained during a puerperal fever autopsy.

Semmelweis had recognized the possibility of person-to-person transmission of an infectious agent. Henceforth he required anyone attending women in labor to scrub their hands with soap, water, and a solution of chlorinated lime. He also limited the number of vaginal examinations during active labor. Strict enforcement of these rules effected dramatic reductions in mortality. Over the next few months, maternal death rates in Semmelweis's ward declined from 18 to about 1 percent!

Nevertheless, in spite of these spectacular results, general reaction to Semmelweis's work was adverse. The majority of the scientific medical establishment continued to attribute puerperal sepsis to miasma (infection through noxious vapors or "bad air"), overcrowding, poor ventilation, or other factors. Not only did Semmelweis's observations conflict with traditional medical thought, but he offered no scientific rationale for his findings. Ultimately, frustrated in his professional ambitions and unable to endure continued "obstinate ignoring of his teachings and the stubborn ruminations of errors," Semmelweis returned to his native Hungary where he continued teaching his methods. He published his findings in his 1861 *Etiology, Concept and Prophylaxis of Childbed Fever.* Sadly, his work did not gain acceptance until after his death. After suffering progressive cognitive decline and mood changes, he was committed to a mental institution in 1865 where he died two weeks later of a gangrenous wound.

Scottish surgeon Joseph Lister was the first to apply effective antiseptic principles to surgical practice. Lister had noticed that most closed fractures—broken bones with intact skin—healed well, but that open fractures—those where bone was exposed—frequently developed purulent infections. Similar complications followed amputations and other operations. In his Male Accident Ward at Glasgow Royal Infirmary, between 1861 and 1865, nearly 50 percent of amputation cases died of sepsis. Rather than accepting the traditional miasmatic explanation, Lister hypothesized that wound sepsis might be due to a pollen-like dust. Having learned of Pasteur's work, he realized that the invisible airborne particles he called "disease dust" were likely similar to the microscopic organisms involved in fermentation. To prevent microbial growth in the operative field, he tried a spray of carbolic acid (phenol, an organic compound that was used to clean foul-smelling sewers), thus establishing an antiseptic barrier between the wound and the germ-containing atmosphere. Instruments and dressings were soaked in dilute carbolic acid, and the surgeon's gown rinsed in the same solution. Lister's results were dramatic: in his ward, from 1865 to 1869, surgical mortality fell by two-thirds to 15 percent.

Once again, initial reception of this new technique was mixed, but over the next decade increasing numbers of surgeons throughout Europe took up Lister's methods. In contrast to Semmelweis, Lister benefited from a scientific climate prepared to accept the concept of microbial agency. His pioneering work was the start of increasingly refined techniques to sterilize the surgical environment. In 1886, steam sterilization was introduced in Berlin. This gradually led to complete asepsis, the technique based on microbial decontamination of everything that comes in contact with the wound. Preoperative scrubbing procedures were augmented in the 20th century, first by the introduction of rubber surgical gloves followed by the addition of the gauze mask. Although Lister's carbolic acid spray is no longer employed today, his principle—rigorous wound disinfection—remains the foundation of modern sterile techniques and surgical antisepsis.

Bibliography and Suggested Readings

Gaynes, Robert P., *Germ Theory: Medical Pioneers in Infectious Diseases*, Washington: ASM Press, 2011.

Larson, Elaine, "Innovations in Health Care: Antisepsis as a Case Study," *American Journal of Public Health* 1989, 79(1): 92–99.

Lister, Joseph, "On the Antiseptic Principle in the Practice of Surgery," *British Medical Journal* 1867, vol. ii: 246, reprinted April 1, 1967, 2(5543): 9–12.

Nuland, Sherwin, *The Doctors' Plague: Germs, Childbed Fever, and the Strange Story of Ignác Semmelweis*, New York: W. W. Norton, 2003.

Semmelweis, Ignaz, *The Etiology, Concept, and Prophylaxis of Childbed Fever*, translated and edited, with an introduction by Carter, K. Codell, Madison: University of Wisconsin Press, 1983.

DNA and the Genetic Code

What	DNA (deoxyribonucleic acid) is the main constituent of chromosomes. Within its structure it stores the genetic code. This code is the biochemical basis of heredity and directs the synthesis of

	specific proteins that determine the characteristics of nearly every living organism.
Where	United Kingdom; United States
When	1953; 1961–1966
By Whom	Francis Crick (1916–2004); Rosalind Franklin (1920–1958); James Watson (1928–); Maurice Wilkins (1916–2004); Robert Holley 1922–1993); Har Gobind Khorana (1922–2011); Marshal Nirenberg (1927–2010); many others
Importance	Revolutionized the field of genetics; ushered in an era where genetic information is used to diagnose and prevent disease, predict disease risk, and develop treatment tailored to the individual.

The discovery of the structure of DNA has been called the most important scientific advance of the 20th century. Considered the "molecule of life," DNA stores the information needed for the cells of nearly every living organism to perform their functions. It is also responsible for the transmission of information to the next generation, the process of heredity.

DNA is made up of building blocks called *nucleotides*, and is a long molecule, or polymer. Each nucleotide contains a sugar (deoxyribose), an organic compound called a *base*, and a phosphate group that links one nucleotide to the next. DNA subunits differ through their bases—adenine, thymine, guanine, and cytosine (abbreviated A, T, G, and C). The structure of DNA consists of two strands of nucleotides twisted around each other in a spiral, ladder-like configuration held together by hydrogen bonds. Its four bases are always arranged in pairs: A pairs only with T, G only with C, making individual chain sequences interdependent, or complementary. Each human cell contains millions of DNA base pairs organized into sections, or genes, packed into 23 pairs of chromosomes.

The idea that individual characteristics or diseases are inherited is ancient, but the actual mechanism of hereditary transmission long remained obscure. DNA itself was first isolated in 1868 by Swiss chemist Friedrich Miescher who extracted the macromolecule from the pus of old surgical bandages. He called it "nuclein" because it was located in the cell nucleus; eventually it was called nucleic acid.

Two years earlier Gregor Mendel, an Austro-Hungarian Augustinian monk, had published his observations on the crossbreeding of pea plants. Believing that many hereditary traits were passed on as discrete units, he established basic rules of genetic transmission, coining the terms "dominant" and "recessive."

At the same time, German biologist Ernst Häckel proposed that living cells transmitted hereditary information via their nucleus. Soon after, chromosomes were found in the cell nucleus, as were the four constituent bases of DNA.

Mendel's work was rediscovered at the turn of the 19th century, and a few years later British biologist William Bateson first introduced the term "genetics." In 1910, American Thomas Hunt Morgan determined the arrangement of genes, as well as the sex-linked determination of certain traits, within the chromosomes of fruit flies. By 1930, DNA and RNA (ribonucleic acid), the two forms of nucleic acid, and deoxyribose, the sugar linking the phosphate and base components of DNA, had been isolated.

Because chromosomes contained proteins and DNA, it was generally believed that genes must be made up of proteins and that they were the transmitters of inheritance, with DNA serving only an ancillary role. The chemical structure of DNA itself was thought too simple to transmit complex information. It was not until 1943 that Rockefeller Institute microbiologist Oswald Avery overturned this theory. He added purified DNA extracted from a pneumococcal culture to a different strain of the bacterium, which resulted in the growth of several stable generations of the initial strain. This demonstrated that contrary to prevailing thought, DNA was the "transforming principle." It meant, Avery wrote, that DNA was "functionally active . . . and that by means of a known chemical substance it [was] possible to induce *predictable and hereditary changes . . . [original emphasis]*"

In 1950 biochemist Erwin Chargaff recognized that the DNA base pairs were present in similar amounts. This paired relationship, "Chargaff's rule," became a key principle for understanding DNA structure. In 1951, American scientist and future Nobel laureate Linus Pauling suggested that the DNA macromolecule might have a helical structure. The same year, James Watson, a young molecular biologist from Chicago, started working with Francis Crick at Cambridge University. The two shared a common interest in DNA and decided to study its configuration using molecular models based on Pauling's work.

In 1952, King's College physicist Maurice Wilkins, who was analyzing the structure of DNA through X-ray diffraction, showed Watson some of his colleague Rosalind Franklin's unpublished data. This proved to be crucial information, leading Watson and Crick to build the now-famous double-helix model of the molecule. Both later acknowledged the importance of Franklin's images in confirming the validity of their helical configuration. Their DNA model, published in April 1953 together with Wilkins's and Franklin's diffraction studies, showed the base pairs A-T and G-C held together by hydrogen bonds inside the helix, with a sugar-phosphate spine outside, and the phosphate molecule linking to the next nucleotide. The complementary pairing of bases on the intertwined chains suggested, as Watson and Crick put forth in their landmark publication, "a possible copying mechanism for genetic material." Indeed, when a cell divides, two strands of complementary DNA separate, with each becoming the template for an identical double helix in the new cell through a process called replication.

In 1962, Watson, Crick, and Wilkins were awarded the Nobel Prize for their discoveries; Franklin, who in 1958 had died of ovarian cancer at age 37, did not qualify for the prize posthumously. But between them, they had uncovered the molecular nature of heredity. Their work marked a turning point in the history of genetics: it was now possible to study how genetic material is stored, replicated, and transmitted from one generation to the next.

However, the exact mechanism of how DNA controls specific amino acid production was as yet unknown. The credit for elucidating this process and "breaking" the genetic code went to American biochemists Marshall Nirenberg, Robert Holley, and Har Gobind Khorana. They were the first to explain the relationship between the information stored in DNA and that contained in protein molecules. In the early 1960s, they showed how a gene (a region of DNA) is transcribed onto RNA molecules, a process that requires three different types of RNA (messenger, transfer, and ribosomal RNA).

The RNA nucleotide sequences, which mirror that of DNA, specify which amino acids are to be incorporated, thus controlling the sequence of amino acids of the protein to be synthesized. Each of the 20 amino acids making up our protein substrate is encoded by a series of three nucleotides known as a "codon"; for example, the DNA codon AAA codes for the amino acid lysine. By 1966, the entire code of all 64 possible triplets and the specific amino acids they encode was deciphered. Holley, Khorana, and Nirenberg were awarded the 1968 Nobel Prize in Physiology or Medicine "for their interpretation of the genetic code and its function in protein synthesis."

Unraveling the genetic code has led to extraordinary technological advances in clinical medicine, medical genetics, molecular biology, and related fields. The genome sequences for many disease-causing viruses, bacteria, and parasites could now be cataloged. Methods were developed to sequence, copy, cleave, and manipulate DNA, allowing production of specific proteins for diagnostic procedures, vaccines, drugs, and gene therapies. DNA-based testing quickly detected pathogens, enabling prompt treatment, and identified new microbial strains, allowing for rapid formulation of vaccines. DNA has been studied as a biomarker for early recognition and treatment monitoring in certain cancers. In prenatal diagnosis, genetic screening locates hereditary diseases through amniocentesis, chorionic villus sampling, and other methods.

DNA-based research has also advanced the understanding of diseases. Many have now been defined as alterations at the chromosomal or nucleic acid level. In the 1980s, cystic fibrosis, Huntington's chorea, and hemophilia were among those recognized as single-gene hereditary disorders. The completion of the Human Genome Project in 2003 and the development of rapid DNA sequencing techniques revealed both the extent of variability in the human genome and many polygenic gene–disease associations. Variability is mostly due to single-nucleotide polymorphisms (SNPs), where a single nucleotide base is at variance, and has led to testing multiple SNPs for association with particular diseases. SNP analysis, together with a technique called genome-wide association studies (GWAS), which compares large groups of patients to healthy individuals, is now helping to pinpoint the genomic basis of common diseases such as diabetes, hypertension, rheumatoid arthritis, and many cancers.

The knowledge gained from genetic analysis can inform many strategic decisions about disease management. Simple dietary supplementation or restriction can reduce or eliminate toxic compounds in conditions such as phenylketonuria or homocystinuria and affect biochemical pathways. Certain genetic characteristics can affect patient response to drugs such as anticoagulants or statins. The great hope is that genomic analysis and gene manipulation will ultimately lead to effective gene therapy, targeting specific defects or alterations. At this time, however, treatments to change gene expression or normalize gene function are still experimental.

Bibliography and Suggested Readings

Acharya, Tara, and Sankaran, Neeraja, *The Human Genome Sourcebook,* Westport: Greenwood Press, 2005.

Hunter, Graeme K., *Vital Forces: The Discovery of the Molecular Basis of Life,* London: Academic Press, 2000.

MacDermot, John, and Kempner, Ellis, "The Interpretation of the Genetic Code," in *Nobel Prizes That Changed Medicine,* ed. G. Thompson, Singapore: World Scientific Publishing Co., 2011, pp. 113–131.

Scott, James, and Thompson, Gilbert, "The Discovery of the Structure of DNA" in *Nobel Prizes That Changed Medicine,* ed. G. Thompson, Singapore: World Scientific Publishing Co., 2011, pp. 89–111.

Watson, James, *The Double Helix,* London: Weidenfeld and Nicolson, 1968.

Germ Theory of Disease

What	Medical theory according to which specific diseases are caused by specific germs, or microorganisms, infecting the body.
Where	Italy; France; Germany
When	1830s to 1880s
By Whom	Agostino Bassi (1773–1856); Louis Pasteur (1822–1895); Robert Koch (1843–1910)
Importance	Revolutionized the understanding of disease mechanisms and brought about lasting change in the practice of medicine; supplanted ancient medical theories of miasma and provided the basis for identifying disease-causing germs and lifesaving treatments; gave birth to microbiology and related fields.

The discovery that bacteria caused disease and were responsible for contagion was unquestionably the most significant medical advance of the 19th century. That certain illnesses might be caused by organisms too small to be seen with the naked eye was not a new idea. As early as the first century B.C. the Roman Marcus Varro warned of swampy areas because they "bred certain minute creatures which cannot be seen . . . but which float in the air and enter the body through the mouth and nose and cause serious diseases." In the 16th century, physician-scholar Girolamo Fracastoro speculated that tiny spores, or "seeds," of disease in the environment were capable of transmitting infection. His treatise *On Contagion and Contagious Diseases* formulated early scientific concepts of the nature of disease germs and their modes of transmission by direct contact or through the air. In 1835 the Italian entomologist Agostino Bassi found that a local silkworm disease was due to a fungal parasite and hypothesized that as yet unknown live organisms might be the cause of such diseases as smallpox, cholera, and plague.

French physicians Casimir Davaine and Pierre Rayer in 1850 were the first to confirm the disease-causing role of microbes with their studies on the nature of the anthrax bacillus. A large, rod-shaped bacterium, anthrax commonly infected sheep and other livestock. By injecting healthy animals with the blood of sick sheep Davaine and Rayer were able not only to reproduce the disease, but also to detect the bacillus in their experimental animals.

But it was largely the groundbreaking work of Louis Pasteur and Robert Koch in the latter half of the 19th century that provided the incontrovertible scientific evidence for the germ theory of disease. Pasteur, who had originally been trained as a chemist, began his biological investigations in the 1850s at the faculty of science at Lille when a local distiller asked him to look into problems with alcoholic fermentation of beet sugar. Until then this process had been assumed to be entirely chemical, with the dying yeast emitting an inert chemical catalyst. Rather than confirming the established view, Pasteur's experiments determined that yeasts bud and multiply during sugar fermentation and that the amount of alcohol produced was directly correlated to the growth of live fungal organisms; these could be cultured and studied in the laboratory. He also found that fermentation failure or spoilage was due to foreign organisms competing with yeast. These unwanted microbes could be destroyed by heat. The process, later called pasteurization, was successfully applied to the making of wine, beer, and vinegar, as well as to the preservation and sterilization of milk. Pasteur's work on diseases of fermentation had far-reaching practical and public health applications.

In later years, these discoveries led Pasteur to investigate infectious diseases in animals and humans, with findings that would revolutionize preventive medicine. While studying the microbes that caused chicken cholera, he observed that cultures grown in a certain temperature range lost their virulence, yet could induce resistance in healthy fowls. In 1881, he tested this method against anthrax, conducting a now-famous public experiment at the village of Pouilly-le-Fort where he inoculated 24 sheep with heat-attenuated bacilli. Another 24 were used as controls. The sheep were then injected with virulent anthrax. The inoculated animals remained healthy, whereas all the others died.

This dramatic experiment established a basic immunological principle: that exposure to attenuated pathogenic organisms would afford protection against the disease caused by this organism. Together with his collaborator Emile Roux, Pasteur went on to develop an attenuated form of the causative agent of rabies, a disease that was invariably fatal. In 1885, using dried, weakened rabies virus he successfully treated nine-year-old Joseph Meister, a young boy who had suffered multiple bites from a rabid dog. He called his new method "vaccination" in tribute to Jenner's previous work.

Meanwhile, Pasteur's younger German contemporary Robert Koch, a country physician and a meticulous investigator, worked on some of the same disease causation problems. Koch may well have been primed for his research by Jacob Henle, his professor and another early proponent of the idea that contagious diseases might be due to living microscopic parasites. In the course of his investigations Koch developed sophisticated techniques for isolating and culturing pathogenic bacteria and perfected methods for staining and even photographing bacteria at a time when improvements in microscopy allowed for increased image resolution and illumination. Thus he gradually succeeded in elucidating the life cycle of the anthrax bacillus and in discovering the causes of a number of infectious diseases, including cholera, sleeping sickness, and, most importantly, tuberculosis. Since then, his four fundamental criteria to prove disease causation and transmission have become universally known as "Koch's postulates." In 1905 Koch was awarded the Nobel Prize "for his investigations and discoveries in relation to tuberculosis."

Both Pasteur and Koch introduced new standards and techniques in scientific research, contributing significantly to the rise of laboratory medicine. What was more, their groundbreaking studies definitively invalidated the previous widely held theories of disease causation through miasma—bad air—or of spontaneous generation—the view that life could arise from inanimate matter as the result of chemical processes. Their work also explained the successful

Koch's Postulates

In 1884 Robert Koch formulated four criteria that he considered the *sine qua non* for establishing a causative relationship between an infectious microbe and a particular disease. To be such a causative agent:

1. a specific microorganism or pathogen must be present in all cases of a given disease
2. the pathogen must be isolated from the diseased host and grown in pure culture
3. the cultured microbe should cause disease when inoculated into a healthy, susceptible organism; and
4. the pathogen must be isolated from the newly infected experimental host and shown to be the same as the originally inoculated pathogen.

These principles have gained scientific and historical recognition as *Koch's postulates*. Although not universally applicable, especially in the setting of viral diseases, they still inform the modern-day approach to microbial diagnosis.

Source: Evans, Alfred, "Causation and Disease: The Henle-Koch Postulates Revisited," *Yale Journal of Biology and Medicine* May 1976, 49 (2): 175–195.

results of Semmelweis's and Lister's antiseptic methods and laid the foundation for the future fields of bacteriology and microbiology. Because infectious disease could now be reduced to specific, perhaps preventable, albeit not yet treatable, causes, old tenets of hygiene and sanitation were reinforced and improved. As bacteriologists identified the microbes responsible for specific diseases, they also paved the way for controlling the spread of contagion within a community with more rational and effective measures. The increased mass communications and advertising of late-19th-century industrialized society further contributed to disseminating and popularizing public health and sanitary guidelines. Even though antibiotics had not yet arrived, validation and acceptance of the germ theory of disease brought about effective preventive measures and opened the door to future lifesaving treatments.

Bibliography and Suggested Readings

Gaynes, Robert P., *Germ Theory: Medical Pioneers in Infectious Diseases*, Washington: ASM Press, 2011.

Geison, Gerald L., *The Private Science of Louis Pasteur*, Princeton: Princeton University Press, 1995.

Porter, Roy, *The Greatest Benefit to Mankind: A Medical History of Humanity from Antiquity to the Present*, London: Harper-Collins, 1997.

Rosen, George, *A History of Public Health*, Baltimore: Johns Hopkins University Press, 2015.

Warner, John Harley, *The Therapeutic Perspective: Medical Practice, Knowledge, and Identity in America*, Cambridge: Harvard University Press, 1986.

Helicobacter Pylori

What	*Helicobacter pylori* is a gram-negative bacterium that infects gastric mucosa; it is the main cause of chronic gastritis and peptic ulcers.
Where	Australia
When	1983
By Whom	J. Robin Warren (1937–), Barry J. Marshall (1951–)
Importance	Revolutionized the understanding of peptic ulcer disease and made it easily curable; helped prevent gastric cancer.

Peptic ulcer disease is one of the most common diseases of mankind, affecting millions of people worldwide. Peptic ulcers are erosions of the gastric or duodenal mucosa, which develop as a result of inflammation. In the acid environment of gastric juice, they persist and, if deep enough, can lead to severe complications, including pain, bleeding, and perforation. In the United States alone, peptic ulcer disease is a major cause of morbidity; in the 1990s associated healthcare costs were estimated at over $5.6 billion annually.

The discovery that a bacterium, *H. pylori*, was at the root of most cases of gastritis (inflammation of the stomach) and peptic ulcer has been called one of the great clinical paradigm shifts in 20th-century medicine. Indeed, until then physicians had considered the stomach a sterile environment, where the acidity of gastric juices would make bacterial survival impossible. Pathologists had occasionally reported the presence of spiral bacteria in gastric specimens, but such findings were dismissed as incidental. For many decades, the idea that ulcers were due to excess acid production engendered by modern-day stress, poor diet, alcohol, and tobacco had prevailed among clinicians and governed their approaches to treatment. The theory that psychological stress caused ulcers arose following animal experiments in which extreme physical stress led to peptic ulcerations; stress ulcers had also been found in burn and other intensive care patients.

Together with pain relief and stress reduction, early treatments of ulcer patients consisted of diet. A hundred years ago, medical textbooks recommended that peptic ulcers be treated with complete rest, food given for a few days entirely by the rectum, then milk every two to three hours "peptonized with 'liquor pancreaticus' "—a concoction of fresh chopped pancreas and dilute alcohol, mixed with boiled milk and bicarbonate of soda. The 1915 "Sippy" diet, devised by Chicago physician Bertram Sippy, was less radical; it consisted of large doses of milk, eggs, and antacids and survived in clinical practice until well into the 1970s when the acid inhibitors known as H2 receptor blockers were first introduced. These drugs were effective, had few side effects, and even though clinical trials showed bismuth (*Pepto-Bismol*) to be equally useful, the H2 antagonists cimetidine (*Tagamet*) and ranitidine (*Zantac*) became so popular that by the 1990s they had become the world's bestselling drugs. None of these therapies were curative, but they bolstered the stress–acid dogma of peptic ulcer disease. Ulcers healed when gastric acid production was inhibited, yet without treatment patients relapsed.

The advent in the 1970s of flexible fiber-optic endoscopy enabled easier visualization of ulcers, as well as demonstration of healing. Technological advances also made possible larger, more targeted stomach biopsies and provided plenty of tissue samples for observation. Pathologists began to notice what appeared to be bacteria in the stomach and duodenum. In 1979, one of them, J. Robin Warren at the Royal Perth Hospital in Western Australia, was studying biopsy tissue from patients with gastritis when he encountered unexpectedly large colonies of spiral-shaped bacteria together with damaged stomach cells.

Over the next two years he collected numerous samples, showing the presence of the same bacteria in many gastric biopsies. They were usually related to chronic gastritis and found grouped under the mucous layer of the stomach; they could therefore not be mouth flora or secondary contaminants. Yet, none of his clinical colleagues were interested in the potential significance of these findings.

In 1981 29-year-old Barry Marshall, training in general medicine, was sent to meet Warren to collect data for a clinical gastroenterology project. Marshall had immediate interest in the possibility that a heretofore-unknown bacterium could be the cause of gastritis and peptic ulceration. An early indication that these bacteria were clinically significant was when a patient with severe gastritis responded to a two-week course of antibiotics. To investigate these findings further, Marshall collected biopsy samples from 13 endoscopy patients; he subsequently expanded his study to 100 patients with gastric inflammation or ulcerations. The organism was present in almost all. Routine tissue cultures of the first 36 samples yielded no results. Number 37, however, inadvertently left in the incubator for five days over a holiday weekend, grew nearly pure *H. pylori* cultures.

In June 1983 Warren and Marshall reported their findings in two letters to the *Lancet*, concluding that if the bacteria observed were "truly associated with . . . gastritis, . . . they may have a part to play in other poorly understood, gastritis-associated diseases." Their insight was prescient. The bacteria were soon shown to cause peptic ulcers. Later epidemiological studies also revealed that persistent infection was a major cause of stomach cancer. The organisms were eventually classified as a new species and named *Helicobacter pylori*, after their corkscrew shape and their site of predilection: the pylorus, the gastric gateway to the small intestine.

At first, the idea that ulcers could be due to a bacterial cause rather than to lifestyle (or to dose-dependent nonsteroidal anti-inflammatories including aspirin, which damage the mucosa by inhibiting prostaglandin synthesis in gastric mucosa) was slow to gain acceptance. Gastroenterologists were skeptical. Infectious disease specialist Martin Blaser, who himself later became a researcher in the field, thought the thing "preposterous" and Marshall "a madman."

Marshall and Warren's work had correlated *H. pylori* infection with gastritis and peptic ulcers. However, in order to establish that *H. pylori* was in fact the cause of the disease, according to Robert Koch's famous postulates, the cultured organism must be shown to induce the disease experimentally. To prove this, Marshall undertook a self-experiment. He started with endoscopic biopsies of his own stomach to prove that his tissue was normal and did not harbor the bacterium. After allowing a month's time for healing, he then swallowed a brew of *H. pylori* in alkaline suspension; he also took cimetidine to inhibit acid production and assist bacterial survival.

After five days, he developed indigestion, nausea, headaches, vomiting, and foul breath. Follow-up gastroscopy and biopsy 10 days after the start of his symptoms showed that he had acute gastritis and that the spiral bacteria had established themselves in his stomach. On the 14th day, Marshall treated himself with tinidazole (an antibiotic) and bismuth, whereupon his symptoms promptly resolved. A final biopsy showed no evidence of *H. pylori*. Clearly, this trial had induced an acute gastric inflammation, supporting the hypothesis that ingestion of *H. pylori* led to infection and secondary gastritis.

Marshall's 1984 self-experiment fostered much interest in his findings. In 1985 he conducted a first randomized controlled trial of antibiotic treatment for ulcers, resulting in eradication of *H. pylori* and marked reduction of ulcer recurrence. Others soon confirmed these findings and helped broaden Marshall's base of investigation. In spite of opposition from various quarters, including suspicious academics and worried pharmaceutical firms (whose now-threatened profits had funded much of contemporary ulcer research), therapeutic practice changed. By 1992, diagnosis of *H. pylori* had become central to ulcer management. By 1994, the World Health Organization (WHO) classified the bacterium as a carcinogen, highlighting its role in gastric cancer.

The most immediate impact of the Australian discovery was on peptic ulcer therapy. For the first time, a condition previously thought to be lifelong could be cured by a short, inexpensive course of treatment. In 2005, Barry J. Marshall and J. Robin Warren were awarded the Nobel Prize in Physiology or Medicine *"for their discovery of the bacterium Helicobacter pylori and its role in gastritis and peptic ulcer disease."* Their work "with tenacity and a prepared mind" had challenged entrenched views and vested interests and transformed the understanding of peptic ulcer disease. Through studies of human volunteers, antibiotic regimens, and epidemiological investigations, it has now been firmly established that *H. pylori* causes more than 90 percent of duodenal ulcers and up to 80 percent of gastric ulcers.

Bibliography and Suggested Readings

Cullingworth, Charles J., *A Manual of Nursing, Medical and Surgical*, London: J & A Churchill, 1883.

Hawkey, Chris, "The Discovery of Helicobacter Pylori," in *Nobel Prizes That Changed Medicine, ed.* Gilbert Thompson, Singapore: World Scientific Publishing Co., 2011, pp. 281–307.

Marshall Barry, and Warren, Robin J., "Unidentified Curved Bacilli on Gastric Epithelium in Active Chronic Gastritis," *Lancet* 1983, 321: 1273–1275.

Meyers, Morton, *Happy Accidents: Serendipity in Modern Medical Breakthroughs,* New York: Arcade Publishing, 2007.

Hepatitis C

What	Identification of hepatitis C virus (HCV) established the cause of infectious hepatitis C.
Where	United States
When	1989
By Whom	Michael Houghton (1949–); Qui-Lim Choo; George Kuo; Harvey Alter (1935–); Daniel W. Bradley (1941–)
Importance	Made possible near-eradication of transfusion-associated hepatitis; led to effective diagnosis and HCV treatment and paved the way for future development of a vaccine.

Hepatitis C is a communicable disease, which affects primarily the liver and is caused by the hepatitis C virus (HCV). The term *hepatitis* simply means liver inflammation; it can have many causes, including alcohol use, drugs or toxins, or infection. Infectious hepatitis usually refers to liver damage produced by one of several viruses. The three major ones identified to date are A, B, and C.

In hepatitis C, early infection is often asymptomatic, but if the condition persists it leads to fibrotic scarring of the liver, and in severe cases to cirrhosis and ultimate liver failure or to hepatocellular cancer. The disease is blood borne and is spread primarily through improperly sterilized medical equipment or by dirty needles used for intravenous drug injection. Before the discovery of the virus, the infection was frequently transmitted via blood transfusions.

Until the 1950s hepatitis had mostly been equated with jaundice, a result of bile duct obstruction or failure of the liver to clear metabolic breakdown products from the blood. Initially only two types of viral hepatitis were thought to exist. They were distinguished on the basis of their incubation periods and epidemiology. However, even after the hepatitis A virus (HAV) and hepatitis B virus (HBV) were identified in the 1960s and 1970s, large numbers of patients were still found to exhibit symptoms such as jaundice or elevated liver enzymes, yet they were not infected by either HAV or HBV. It was therefore postulated that they harbored another infection, originally classified only as non-A non-B (NANB) hepatitis.

It had been known for many years that blood products could transmit hepatitis. These dangers had become starkly obvious when during World War II an estimated 50,000 U.S. soldiers developed hepatitis after inoculation with hepatitis-contaminated yellow fever vaccine; the implicated vaccine lots were subsequently withdrawn and replaced with vaccine free of human serum. At the same time, together with the increasingly widespread use of therapeutic blood transfusion, viral hepatitis began to be recognized as one of its major complications. The first case reports of seven patients who developed jaundice one to four weeks after transfusion with blood or plasma were published in 1943. In that era, viral hepatitis was still believed to be limited to so-called "infectious hepatitis" (A) and "serum hepatitis" (B). Transfusion-associated disease was attributed to hepatitis B.

In the 1970s, U.S. hematologist Harvey Alter at the National Institutes of Health (NIH) and his research team at the Department of Transfusion Medicine began studying post-transfusion hepatitis. They established early on improved criteria for diagnosis of viral hepatitis, which included repeated screening for elevated liver enzymes whether the patient was jaundiced or not. Prior to this, diagnosis had been based largely on development of jaundice, which in most cases of hepatitis C does not occur. Alter had also carefully collected blood samples from both transfusion recipients and their blood donors and had developed a detailed, well-documented repository. In 1973, by which time both hepatitis A and B viruses had been identified, retrospective serological study of his stored blood samples revealed that only about 25 percent of transfusion hepatitis cases were attributable to HBV and none to HAV. This led investigators to attribute the remaining cases to so-called "non-A non-B" hepatitis, which was also infectious, for it was experimentally transmissible to chimpanzees.

Early efforts by Alter's team at NIH and researchers at the Centers for Disease Control and Transmission (CDC) failed to identify the NANB virus, but eventually a screening strategy of viral DNA clones bore fruit. Spearheading the discovery was British scientist Michael Houghton who in 1982 had been recruited by California biotechnology firm Chiron to work on identifying the NANB hepatitis virus associated with post-transfusion hepatitis. By 1987, after various unsuccessful approaches to find and culture the virus, Houghton and his collaborators Qui-Lim Choo and George Kuo, together with Daniel Bradley at the CDC, had elaborated a new molecular cloning method aiming to isolate the virus. Rather than a complementary nucleic acid probe, this method used cloned antibody, presumed specific, derived from serum of a patient with highly active liver disease, to screen for the presence of viral antigen. After screening multiple test samples, one small antibody clone finally succeeded in identifying the virus: it reacted only with infected, not uninfected, sera. Houghton and his colleagues had thus proved the existence of a third agent, a single-stranded RNA virus with a lipid envelope, classified as a *flavivirus*. They named it hepatitis C virus. Their clone was ultimately used to define and sequence the entire viral genome and to create a new diagnostic assay, an antibody test for the virus.

The following year, in 1988, Alter confirmed the presence of the same virus in a series of NANB hepatitis blood samples among the stores he had assembled from both donor and recipient material earlier. The investigators' conclusion, published in 1989, was that the newly discovered hepatitis C virus was a major cause of non-A non-B hepatitis throughout the world.

In 1990, the United States introduced mandatory HCV testing of the blood supply, and by 1992 blood banks had eliminated HCV from their supplies. As a result, the incidence of transfusion-associated hepatitis fell from 30 percent in 1970 to virtually zero. In addition, new serological tests allowed further study of the natural history of the disease. They have established that chronic hepatitis C is one of the most common causes of cirrhosis and chronic liver disease, affecting an estimated 170 million people throughout the world. Hepatitis C has a mortality rate ranging from 1–5 percent; it is the leading indication for liver transplantation.

Houghton and Alter's discovery of the hepatitis C virus was a major biomedical breakthrough that led not only to significant advances in the diagnosis and prevention of liver disease, but also to new antiviral treatments. In 2000, both scientists were honored with the prestigious Lasker Award for their pioneering work.

Today, the blood supply is safer than ever before. The entire genome of the hepatitis C virus has been sequenced. Specific polymerase chain reaction (PCR) assays are used to tailor treatment of hepatitis C disease. Although no HCV vaccine is available yet, new virus culture methods have resulted in specific antiviral therapies that inhibit viral replication and offer the promise of definitive cure.

Bibliography and Suggested Readings

Black, Francis, "Infectious Hepatitis," in *The Cambridge World History of Human Disease*, ed. Kenneth F. Kiple, Cambridge: Cambridge University Press: 1993, pp. 794–799.

Centers for Disease Control and Prevention, 2016, "Hepatitis C FAQs for the Public," http://www.cdc.gov/hepatitis/hcv/cfaq.htm.

Choo, Qui-Lim, Kuo, George, Weiner, Amy J., Overby, Lacy R., Bradley, Daniel W., and Houghton, Michael, "Isolation of a cDNA Clone Derived from a Blood-Borne Non-A, Non-B Viral Hepatitis Genome," *Science* April 21, 1989; 244(4902): 359–362.

Houghton, Michael, "Discovery of the Hepatitis C Virus," *Liver International* January 2009, 29: 82–88.

Seeff, Leonard, and Ghany, Marc, "Harvey Alter and Michael Houghton: The Discovery of Hepatitis C and the Introduction of Screening to Prevent Its Transmission in Transfused Blood," in *Pioneers of Medicine Without a Nobel Prize*, ed. G. Thompson, London: Imperial College Press, 2014, pp. 197–213.

Taylor, Milton W., "Hepatitis" in *Viruses and Man: A History of Interactions*, Switzerland: Springer International Publishing, 2014.

Human Papilloma Virus

What	Small double-stranded DNA virus that can cause abnormal growth of skin and other cells. Long-standing infection with certain human papilloma virus (HPV) types can lead to cancer, especially of the cervix. HPV also causes certain anal, vaginal, vulvar, penile, oropharyngeal, and squamous cell skin cancers.
Where	Germany; Australia; United States
When	1984; 1991; 1993
By Whom	Harald zur Hausen (1936–); Ian Frazer (1953–); Jian Zhou (1957–1999); Douglas Lowy (1942–); John Schiller (1953–)
Importance	Revolutionized prevention strategies through HPV testing and vaccination; development of prophylactic HPV vaccines now permits effective prevention of HPV-induced cervical and related cancers.

The human papilloma virus, or HPV, has been firmly established as the major cause of cervical cancer, the second most common cancer in women. Worldwide, more than half a million women are diagnosed with cervical cancer every year. Over half of them will die of the disease. Most cases and deaths occur in developing countries.

Today, over 120 different HPV types have been identified and classified into low-risk or high-risk subtypes. Low-risk subtypes cause benign skin or mucosal growths such as warts, including genital warts. High-risk subtypes, on the other hand, can induce malignant neoplasms of the genital tract and other sites, primarily the mucosa of the oral cavity and anus. The most common oncogenic HPV types are 16, 18, 31, and 33; they are the ones most prominently responsible for cancers of the cervix, vagina, vulva, penis, anus, and oropharynx. HPV 16 and 18 cause approximately 70 percent of all cervical cancers.

HPV is highly contagious, with an estimated per-partner transmission probability of 60 percent. It is considered the world's most common sexually transmitted infection, with rates increasing steadily since the 1970s and global prevalence estimated at nearly 300 million women.

Warty tumors were described in ancient medical texts, and physicians long ago wrote of skin and genital warts as morbid outgrowths that were potentially contagious. Sexual contact was thought to be a factor. Genital warts were considered the result of sexual promiscuity; perianal warts were associated with homosexual activity. Treatment included topical astringents and surgical excision. In early women's medicine, a popular 12th-century compendium known as the *Trotula* recommended using "a needle [to] lift them up all around. Afterward . . . apply slaked lime . . . and remove them."

In 1842 Verona physician Domenico Rigoni-Stern, an early proponent of medical statistics who had analyzed demographic data in cancer deaths from 1760 to 1839, noted the rare occurrence of cancers of the womb in "single women including nuns." Contrasted to 333 deaths of such cancers in married and widowed women, there were only 20 deaths in the former group, which was presumably sexually inactive. Rigoni-Stern was at a loss to explain this discrepancy, but did not think that cancer could have developed as a result of "mechanical damage."

The infectious nature of common warts was demonstrated in 1907 when Italian physician Ciuffo showed that injection of a cell-free wart extract could induce new growths in uninfected skin. Genital warts were also found to be transmissible, and in 1934 Rockefeller virologists Richard Shope and Peyton Rous showed that papilloma viruses of cottontail rabbits had carcinogenic potential. In 1949 electron microscopy demonstrated the existence of viral particles in the nuclei of epidermal cells of rabbit papillomas.

The DNA structure of human papilloma virus was characterized in 1965. The same year virologists discovered that viral DNA extracted from warts induced skin cancer in rabbits. However, the exact mechanism by which such papilloma-related diseases arose remained unknown. Unlike many other DNA viruses, HPV was difficult to grow in cell culture, for its reproductive cycle depended on differentiated host epithelium. Early research relied heavily on cloning and sequencing of HPV from natural infections, because only a few viral particles could be isolated from patient specimens. Thus it was not until the 1970s, when recombinant DNA technology allowed detailed analysis of the HPV genome, that it became clear there were multiple HPV genotypes.

German virologist Harald zur Hausen was the first to describe various viral strains using transcribed viral RNA and DNA from cutaneous, genital, and cervical cancer biopsies. Having observed striking epidemiological correlations between cervical cancers and genital warts, he considered that the cancer might arise from such infections and postulated the existence of an oncogenic HPV strain. To prove his hypothesis, in 1972 he initiated a series of studies during which he eventually identified a heterogeneous family of HPV viruses, some of which were carcinogenic.

DNA of HPV genotype 6 was found in biopsies of giant *Condylomata acuminata* genital warts; these invasive growths, however, do not metastasize. Shortly after, Hauser and his team succeeded in isolating DNA of HPV 16 and HPV 18 directly from cervical cancer biopsies, as well as from cervical cancer–derived cell lines (including *HeLa* cells). The same year they demonstrated HPV 16 DNA in precursor lesions of anogenital cancers and cervical intraepithelial neoplasias (CINs). In 1992, global epidemiological studies identified HPV 16 and 18, the two most prevalent high-risk genotypes, as the major risk factors for cervical cancer, for they were consistently identified in about 70 percent of all cervical cancer biopsies. Today, there is scientific evidence to link the same types to as many as half of other anogenital cancers, and 25–30 percent of head and neck cancers. Hence HPV turned out to be an important human carcinogen.

The discovery that high-risk strains of HPV were the cause of most invasive cervical cancers led to widespread preventive efforts and spurred massive growth in HPV research. Sequencing of HPV DNA, together with new genetic technologies, helped elucidate the molecular mechanisms of HPV-induced carcinogenesis. In the late 1980s and early 1990s the specific pathways in the malignant transformation of cells by viral oncogenes were defined: HPV itself did not replicate in tumor cells, but certain viral genes were integrated into the cervical cell genome; this foreign DNA, over time, was what reprogrammed cells to grow uncontrollably. In 2008, Harald zur Hausen was awarded the Nobel Prize in Physiology or Medicine "for his discovery of human papilloma viruses causing cervical cancer."

Zur Hausen's groundbreaking work was critical for the prevention and treatment of HPV disease and led to the development of a vaccine to prevent HPV infection and persistence. A first vaccine was pioneered in 1991 by Australian immunologists Ian Frazer and Jian Zhou. Because HPV viral genomes contained oncogenes, a live attenuated or inactivated vaccine could itself induce cancer. They therefore focused on a subunit approach and used noninfectious but highly immunogenic virus-like particles (VLPs) composed of viral capsid proteins but structurally different from infectious HPV. In 1993, Douglas Lowy and John Schiller at the U.S. National Cancer Institute generated VLPs with greater affinity for HPV, which ultimately served as the basis for the HPV 16 component of the vaccine.

There are currently two HPV vaccines on the market, Gardasil and Cervarix, approved by the U.S. Food and Drug Administration (FDA) in 2006 and 2007. They are type specific, but have some activity against closely related viral genotypes. Both vaccines provide over 95 percent protection against sexually transmitted genotypes, primarily HPV 16 and 18, which cause 70 percent of cervical cancers as well as other genital cancers; Gardasil also prevents most genital warts. The vaccines are safe and effective and confer protection against persistent infection and precancerous lesions. They are also expected to protect against HPV-induced oral cancers.

It is estimated that more than 5 percent of cancers worldwide are due to persistent infection with HPV. Cervical cancer alone is responsible for a significant disease burden, and HPV is present in nearly 100 percent of cases. If implemented widely, vaccination may prevent and perhaps eradicate cervical cancer worldwide.

Bibliography and Suggested Readings

Ault, Kevin A., "Epidemiology and Natural History of Human Papillomavirus Infections in the Female Genital Tract," *Infectious Diseases in Obstetrics and Gynecology* 2006 (Suppl. 2006), 40470: 1–5.

Centers for Disease Control and Prevention, 2015, "Human Papillomavirus (HPV)," http://www.cdc.gov/hpv.

DiMaio, Daniel, "Nuns, Warts, Viruses, and Cancer," *The Yale Journal of Biology and Medicine* 2015, 88(2): 127–129.

National Cancer Institute, 2015, "Human Papillomavirus (HPV) Vaccines," http://www .cancer.gov/about-cancer/causes-prevention/risk/infectious-agents/hpv-vaccine -fact-sheet.

Radosevich, James, ed., *HPV and Cancer*, Dordrecht: Springer Netherlands, 2012.

Rosenblatt, Alberto, and Gustavo de Campos Guidi, Homero, *Human Papillomavirus: A Practical Guide for Urologists*, Berlin, Heidelberg: Springer, 2009.

Schiffman, Mark, et al., "Human Papillomavirus and Cervical Cancer," *Lancet* 2007, 370(9590): 890–907.

Skloot, Rebecca, *The Immortal Life of Henrietta Lacks*, New York: Crown Publishers, 2010.

Wailoo, Keith, Livingston, Julie, Epstein, Steven, and Aronowitz, Robert, eds., *Three Shots at Prevention: The HPV Vaccine and the Politics of Medicine's Simple Solutions*, Baltimore: Johns Hopkins University Press, 2010.

Yanofsky, Valerie, et al., "Genital Warts: A Comprehensive Review," *Journal of Clinical and Aesthetic Dermatology* June 2012, 5(6): 25–36.

zur Hausen, Harald, "Papillomaviruses in the Causation of Human Cancers—A Brief Historical Account," *Virology* 2009, 384(2): 260–265.

Iodine

What	Iodine is an essential micronutrient required for thyroid hormone synthesis. Proper function of the thyroid is critical to normal growth and metabolism of the body, and to maturation of the brain and central nervous system in infants and the young.
Where	France; Switzerland; England; United States
When	19th and early 20th centuries
By Whom	Bernard Courtois (1777–1838); Theodor Kocher (1841–1917); Victor Horsley (1857–1916); Eugen Baumann (1846–1896); David Cowie (1872–1940); many others
Importance	Salt iodization has dramatically reduced iodine deficiency disorders such as goiter throughout the world.

The thyroid gland, a butterfly-shaped organ at the base of the neck, was known in antiquity but its physiological function was not. Some thought it lubricated the voice and larynx, others that it beautified the female neck. The thyroid frequently exhibited pathological changes but its role remained mysterious. Nineteenth-century scientists were the first to hypothesize that it was a gland whose secretions entered the bloodstream.

Goiter was one of the most common disorders affecting the thyroid. An abnormal enlargement of the gland, goiters were endemic in mountainous and landlocked regions and were often associated with severe mental retardation or cretinism. Enlarged glands could also exert pressure on the neighboring trachea or esophagus and interfere with breathing or swallowing. Seaweed and burnt sponge as treatment for goiter had been tried in China as early as 3600 B.C. These remedies appeared to be effective; their continued use was documented in ancient Greek, Roman, and medieval medical texts.

The advent of anesthesia and asepsis in the late 19th century brought attempts at surgical goiter therapy. However, removal of the gland was not a cure. Animal experiments undertaken by German physiologist Moritz Schiff showed complete thyroidectomy to be fatal. In 1883, Theodor Kocher, professor at Bern, found that extirpating the thyroid in man led to numerous abnormalities. Other surgeons observed similar symptoms: lethargy, muscle weakness, limb and facial swelling, anemia, neurological disturbances, and finally death. The syndrome, which Kocher had termed "cachexia strumipriva," was also known as myxedema and was associated with severe goiters. This work established the critical role of the thyroid gland: it acted by producing a vital internal secretion, and in order for surgery to be successful, a functioning portion of the gland must be left in place. Kocher's investigations into the causes and treatment of endemic goiter led to his award in 1909 of the Nobel Prize in Physiology or Medicine *"for his work on the physiology, pathology and surgery of the thyroid gland."*

Meanwhile, between 1884 and 1886, Victor Horsley's experiments in London proved that myxedema, cretinism, and cachexia strumipriva were one and the same. All were brought on by the destruction or degeneration of the thyroid and responded to treatment with extracts of the gland. In 1891, his colleague George Murray reported encouraging results after treating a middle-aged myxedematous woman with extract of sheep thyroid, confirming that the gland played an important metabolic role. Because sluggish growth and poor intellect were associated with goiters, it became fashionable to treat retarded children and even obese or depressed adults with thyroid extract prepared from dried pig or beef glands. Dessicated thyroid extract is still available today.

In 1895 German chemist Eugen Baumann discovered the presence of iodine in the thyroid, suggesting that iodine deficiency was responsible for overgrowth of thyroid tissue. Dietary supplementation could remedy this and thus make possible a cure for goiter. Iodine itself, a trace element mostly present in the soil and water of coastal areas, had not been discovered until 1811 when French chemist Bernard Courtois isolated it during the manufacture of gunpowder. Shortly thereafter, Swiss physician J. F. Coindet had reported that oral administration of grains of iodine decreased the size of his patients' goiters; William Prout in England had proposed the same treatment. In 1852, French scientist Adolphe Chatin had first published the idea of iodine deficiency associated with endemic (geographically localized) goiter.

Baumann's investigations later identified an organic substance, "thyroiodine," of which iodine was an essential constituent. This was thyroxine, the active hormone secreted by the thyroid gland. We now know that if dietary iodine intake is insufficient, the thyroid will not be able to make thyroxine. Hypothyroid endemic—also called simple or colloid—goiter is but the result of negative endocrine feedback on the pituitary gland leading to increased production of TSH (thyroid-stimulating hormone); this in turn causes the thyroid to enlarge in order to compensate for the deficiency and absorb more iodine.

Systematic iodine supplementation—largely through adding iodine to table salt, an inexpensive and universally available food—did not begin until the early 1920s. It was first instituted in Switzerland and in the United States. Prior to this iodine deficiency was widespread in many Alpine regions in Europe. It was also common in the Great Lakes, Appalachian, and Northwestern regions of the United States, a geographic area known as the "goiter belt" where iodine was markedly deficient in water and soil and where large numbers of children and adults had clinically apparent goiter. World

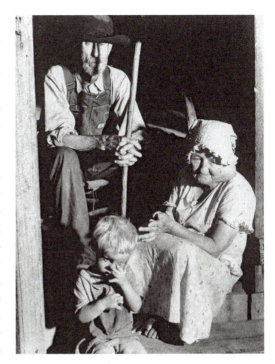

Elderly sharecropper couple with their grandson during the Great Depression, in Sweetfern, Arkansas, 1936. A large goitrous growth disfigures the woman's face and neck. Arkansas was part of the Appalachian "goiter belt" where iodine deficiency in water and soil led to frequent thyroid disease and endemic goiter in children and adults. (Margaret Bourke-White/The LIFE Images Collection/Getty Images)

War I draft physicals in Michigan and later surveillance studies demonstrated a greater than 60 percent prevalence of goiter in certain areas. In 1917, Ohio physician David Marine initiated the first iodine prophylaxis program in schoolgirls and reported a striking decrease in the incidence of goiter in children who were treated. Swiss and Italian investigators four years later obtained similar therapeutic results.

These successes inspired Michigan pediatrician David Cowie to argue for the implementation of statewide prophylaxis modeled on a program instituted in 1922 by the Swiss Goiter Commission, the first to add a specific amount of sodium iodide or potassium iodide to table salt. Cowie's efforts and the work of the Michigan Iodized Salt Committee were instrumental in the introduction of iodine supplementation across the nation in 1924 and the subsequent near-complete eradication of simple goiter in the United States.

Since then, many countries have adopted mandatory iodization of all food-grade salt. In the United States, iodine fortification of salt remains voluntary, and the Food and Drug Administration (FDA) does not mandate listing of iodine content on food packaging. A 1948 bill by the U.S. Endemic Goiter Committee proposing mandatory introduction of iodized salt in all states was defeated. The proportion of U.S. households using iodized salt is currently estimated at 70–76 percent.

Worldwide, iodine deficiency remains an important cause of goiter. Goitrous disease still exists in the Andes and the Himalayas, in part of the European Alps, the highlands of New Guinea, some areas of China, and places where naturally occurring iodine is nutritionally inadequate or where iodide prophylaxis has not reached the population. Almost invariably the iodine levels of these populations are considerably below normal. The World Health Organization maintains a global database on iodine deficiency, including data by country on goiter prevalence and urinary iodine concentrations.

In today's developed world endemic goiter is rare. A hundred years ago it was, in David Marine's words, "one of the most important and widespread causes of human suffering and of physical and mental degeneracy." Understanding the important nutritional role of iodine in preventing this disease was a major public health milestone. Iodine deficiency disease was among the first significant disorders of micronutrient malnutrition to be recognized and treated. The corrective dietary strategies implemented as a result contributed significantly to the development of modern scientific medicine and nutrition.

Bibliography and Suggested Readings

"The Iodine Deficiency Disorders," 2014, http://www.thyroidmanager.org/chapter/the-iodine-deficiency-disorders/#toc-introduction.

Leung, Angela M., Braverman, Lewis E., and Pearce, Elizabeth N., "History of U.S. Iodine Fortification and Supplementation," *Nutrients* 2012, 4(11): 1740–1746.

MacNalty, Arthur, "Sir Victor Horsley: His Life and Work," *British Medical Journal* April 20, 1957, 1(5024): 910–916.

Marine, David, "Etiology and Prevention of Simple Goiter," *Medicine* 1924, 3: 453–479.

Markel, Howard, "'When It Rains It Pours': Endemic Goiter, Iodized Salt, and David Murray Cowie, MD," *American Journal of Public Health* February 1987, 77(2): 219–229.

Porter, Roy, *The Greatest Benefit to Mankind,* Hammersmith, London: Harper Collins, 1997.

Shrady, George F., ed., "The Physiology and Surgery of the Thyroid Gland," *The Medical Record* 1885, 27: 127–128.

World Health Organization, "Micronutrient Deficiencies: Iodine Deficiency Disorders," http://www.who.int/nutrition/topics/idd/en.

Malaria

What	Infectious disease caused by microbial parasites of the genus *Plasmodium*, and transmitted between human hosts by the bite of infected mosquitoes.
Where	Algeria; India; Italy
When	1880; 1897
By Whom	Alphonse Laveran (1845–1922); Ronald Ross (1857–1932); Giovanni Battista Grassi (1854–1925)
Importance	Discovery of the malaria parasite and of its mode of transmission laid the foundation for preventing spread and effectively combating the disease.

An ancient scourge, malaria has persisted as a major public health problem into the 21st century. Despite considerable efforts at eradication the disease continues to affect millions of people throughout the world, mostly in poor tropical regions. Malaria—from the Italian *"mal(a) aria,"* bad air—refers to early associations with miasmatic theories of disease and the noxious emanations of swamps or marshlands, breeding grounds for mosquitoes. For many centuries the disease had been known as paludism, or marsh fever. Its symptoms were documented in ancient Chinese medical treatises and were well recognized in Hippocratic times. Variably attributed to the bite of insects or to stagnant waters, malarial disease remained endemic in parts of Europe and the southeastern United States until the late 1940s.

Malaria is transmitted by the bite of female *Anopheles* mosquitoes, which introduce the malaria parasites from their saliva into the victims' bloodstream. There are several pathogenic species of the malarial protozoan, *Plasmodium*, of which *P. falciparum* is the most virulent. Infected individuals develop paroxysmal fevers, chills, sweats, headaches, and fatigue. Febrile crises typically occur at two- or three-day intervals; they are the "tertian" or "quartan" fevers already described by Hippocrates in the fourth century B.C. Severe cases lead to jaundice, seizures, and death. In survivors, the infection produces a partial resistance to reinfection that will wane with time. There is to date no vaccine.

The question of the nature of malaria, its cause and mode of transmission, and the hope of treating and preventing this disease had long occupied investigators. In the early 17th century New World explorers brought back to Europe an Inca remedy made from the bark of the Peruvian cinchona tree, which provided relief from certain fevers. Its specific therapeutic action allowed physicians to begin to define malaria as a separate clinical entity, distinct from other febrile illnesses. Quinine, the active ingredient of cinchona bark, was isolated in 1820 and is still used as an antimalarial, either alone or in combination with other drugs.

The cause of malaria was not elucidated until 1880 when C. L. Alphonse Laveran, a French army surgeon working at a military hospital in Algeria, first observed a form of the malarial parasite in fresh blood smears of malaria patients. In 1882 he carried out additional studies in Italy on patients suffering from marsh fever, and in 1884 published his *Traité des fièvres palustres* where he described 480 cases of malaria. Laveran found that the parasites responsible for marsh fever destroyed their host's red blood cells. Even though he was unable to demonstrate the existence of the infectious agent outside the patient's body, he hypothesized that it underwent part of its development in mosquitoes, which then served as vectors for transmission. In 1907, Laveran was awarded the Nobel Prize in Physiology or Medicine "in recognition of his work on the role played by protozoa in causing diseases."

Subsequent research led to the identification of distinct developmental forms of the malarial parasite in the bloodstream, each corresponding to different disease stages and explaining the relationships between parasite and red blood cell hosts. Italian scientist Camillo Golgi, famous for his work on the structure of the nervous system, studied plasmodial multiplication and showed that the periodicity of malarial crises was correlated to the appearance of successive new generations of parasites in the patient's blood.

In 1897, British army surgeon Ronald Ross succeeded in demonstrating the role played by the mosquito as both malaria host and vector of disease. His mentor Patrick Manson, an avid student of tropical diseases, had earlier postulated that malarial infections were mosquito borne. Ross in turn, upon entering the Indian Medical Service, undertook to test Manson's hypothesis. Experimenting with mosquitoes hatched in his laboratory at Secunderabad, he had the insects feed on the blood of malaria patients; he then dissected them to look for the parasite, the organism that Laveran had observed. His investigations finally bore fruit when he discovered in the stomach wall of a mosquito several clusters of black granules: they were the eggs described by Laveran, which represented the intermediate stage of the *Plasmodium* life cycle. He thus confirmed Laveran's findings. In subsequent studies Ross demonstrated the development of the parasite within the body of the mosquito: first, as a zygote in its stomach, then as an oocyst (egg) in the stomach lining, and finally as a sporozoite (an immature form of the parasite), which is inoculated into a host through the insect proboscis when it bites and squirts its saliva prior to sucking blood.

At the same time in Italy, physician Giovanni Battista Grassi had independently shown the link between human malaria and the *Plasmodium* parasite by demonstrating how the *Anopheles* mosquito was infected by feeding off the blood of a malaria patient. In 1897, together with collaborators Bignami and Bastianelli, he established the developmental stages of malaria parasites in anopheline mosquitoes; the following year they described the complete life cycles of *P. falciparum*, *P. vivax,* and *P. malariae*, all vectors of human malaria. Noting that not all mosquito-infested areas were malarial, Grassi also recognized that only certain *Anopheles* mosquito species carried the disease.

Ronald Ross was awarded the 1902 Nobel Prize for Physiology or Medicine for his work on malaria, which "laid the foundation for successful research on this disease and methods of combating it." Even though Grassi—who between 1901 and 1925 received 21 nominations for the prize—was first to recognize *Anopheles* as the vector of transmission (Ross had only identified the mosquito as "grey with dappled wings") and by 1898 had described three of the four agents of human malaria, Ross claimed priority and ultimately won the Nobel Committee's support as sole award recipient. The bitter controversy that ensued, documented in published letters between Ross and Grassi, has been the subject of scientific and historical inquiry, including a fictional dramatization in Paul De Kruif's famous *Microbe Hunters* (to which Ross reportedly took exception; as a result, De Kruif's chapter on malaria was deleted in the British edition of the book).

The groundbreaking discovery of the malaria parasite opened the prospect for large-scale disease prevention through control of mosquitoes. In the early 20th century the U.S. Public Health Service, with the support of the Rockefeller Foundation, initiated a variety of antimalarial programs in the southern states with spectacular results, essentially eliminating malaria in the United States. Similar control measures implemented by the Fascist regime in the late 1920s and early 1930s succeeded in eradicating disease in the malarial regions of Italy. These successes encouraged broader measures: after World War II the World Health Organization (WHO) launched a global malaria eradication program, which included draining of swamps, spraying powerful DDT insecticides, and immunizing with chloroquine. Unfortunately, mosquitoes and plasmodia eventually became resistant to these chemical control measures; DDT was banned due to environmental and health concerns. Since 1980 prevention has focused on the use of long-lasting mosquito nets, insect repellents, and indoor residual spraying, as well as pharmacological prophylaxis for dwellers or travellers in endemic areas.

In 2015 malaria is a preventable and treatable disease. Yet, in 2014, the WHO reported for the prior year an estimated 200 million cases of malaria worldwide, with an estimated 584,000 deaths. Ninety percent of all malaria fatalities occurred in Africa; in 2013, approximately 440,000 African children died of malaria before their fifth birthday.

Bibliography and Suggested Readings

Bynum, William F., and Overy, Caroline, eds., *The Beast in the Mosquito: The Correspondence of Ronald Ross and Patrick Manson.* Clio Medica, 51, Wellcome Institute Series in the History of Medicine, Amsterdam: Editions Rodopi, 1998.

Centers for Disease Control and Prevention, 2016, "The History of Malaria, an Ancient Disease," http://www.cdc.gov/malaria/about/history/index.html.

Cook, Gordon, "Ronald Ross (1857–1932): The Role of the Italian Malariologists, and Scientific Verification of Mosquito Transmission of Malaria," in *Tropical Medicine: An Illustrated History of the Pioneers*, Amsterdam, Paris, Boston: Elsevier Academic Press, 2007, pp. 81–102.

Dunn, Frederick L., "Malaria," in *The Cambridge World History of Human Disease*, ed. Kenneth F. Kiple, Cambridge: Cambridge University Press, 2015, pp. 855–862.

Erling, Norrby, *Nobel Prizes and Life Sciences*, Singapore: World Scientific Publishing Co., 2010.

"Nomination Database," 2014, http://www.nobelprize.org/nomination/archive/list.php.

Porter, Roy, *The Greatest Benefit to Mankind: A Medical History of Humanity from Antiquity to the Present,* London: Harper Collins, 1997.

World Health Organization, 2014, "Fact Sheet on the World Malaria Report 2014," http://www.who.int/malaria/media/world_malaria_report_2014/en.

Monoclonal Antibodies

What	Identical antibody molecules produced by a single immune cell clone and binding to the same antigen.
Where	United Kingdom
When	1975

By Whom   César Milstein (1927–2002); Georges Köhler (1946–1995)
Importance   Helped elucidate complex immune mechanisms; provided new
               biomedical tools with vast applications in diagnostics, therapeu-
               tics, and targeted drug delivery systems; in prevention and
               detection of disease; in vaccine production; and in the study of
               genetic disease susceptibility.

The discovery of monoclonal antibodies was the result of a long scientific quest to explain the workings of the immune system, particularly the generation and functional specificity of antibodies, essential to the immune response. The most important task of the immune system is to defend the body against disease-causing germs—bacteria, viruses, and other microbes. Specialized white blood cells called B-lymphocytes are vital in this process. They produce large, Y-shaped protein molecules known as antibodies, or immunoglobulins, to operate an intricate detection system and to identify and neutralize foreign substances or antigens.

Most animals make many different antibodies to fight foreign antigens. As was first demonstrated with human blood group antigens, these antibodies have a very close affinity for individual inciting antigens. This affinity becomes greater the more antigenic substances the immune system is exposed to. Antibodies bind to a specific portion of an antigen called *epitope*, which itself consists of a defined sequence of amino acids. In immune surveillance, antibodies function as veritable scouts, marking the antigen, or antigen–antibody complex, for ultimate destruction by phagocytes.

Monoclonal antibodies are antibodies that bind to a specific antigen epitope and are produced from a single B-lymphocyte clone, derived from one particular cell. Each B-cell, or cell line, can produce only one particular antibody, which in turn recognizes and binds to only one specific antigen. Upon encountering an antigen, a single B-cell or clone of cells will divide to produce many activated B-cells. Most differentiate into plasma cells secreting antibodies to bind the same epitope that elicited their proliferation in the first place; a few survive as memory cells that can recognize only the same, original epitope. Antigenic specificity is an important feature of this immune memory. It explains, in part, how individuals can make so many different antibodies to any given antigen. The effectiveness of the immune response is made possible by the existence of millions of different clones, each one possessing specific antigenic affinity.

It follows that the ability to design "rare antibodies with a tailor-made-like fit for a given structure" and to produce them in large quantities would revolutionize the field of immunology. German scientist Paul Ehrlich, in the early 1900s, had first proposed the idea of a "magic bullet"—a compound that would deliver a specific toxin to target a disease or kill disease-causing cells but leave normal cells unharmed. With Ehrlich's help, Behring and Kitasato's diphtheria antitoxin became the original biological weapon: immune serum antibodies for therapeutic use. Until the late 1930s and the advent of sulfon-amides, serum therapy was used widely for various bacterial diseases, including diphtheria, meningitis, and pneumonia. However, nonhuman antisera could also cause serum sickness, the potentially fatal allergic reaction to foreign immu-nogenic proteins. It would take several more decades for scientists to develop more specific immune substances that would precisely target disease on the cellular level.

Cambridge biochemists César Milstein and Georges Köhler, in 1975, were the first to do so. They produced monoclonal antibodies (mAbs) *in vitro*. Each had been working on antibody production in the laboratory, trying to create long-lived cells that would generate a particular antibody in large quantities. Together, they succeeded in developing a technique where they fused normal antibody-producing B-lymphocytes with cells of multiple myeloma; there were cancerous B-cells that grew and multiplied forever and had the capacity to secrete large amounts of immunoglobulin. The result was a hybrid cell, referred to as *hybridoma*, which not only was immortal but also could secrete a spe-cific antibody.

Milstein and Köhler's hybridoma technique consisted of immunizing mice against a specific antigen and harvesting the immunized B-lymphocytes from the animals' spleen. These were then fused with an immortal myeloma cell line and cultured in a selective medium that allowed only the fused hybrid cells to grow. Individual B-lymphocyte clones were isolated and screened for the specific antibody activity required; those were grown, recloned, and retested for their antigen-binding activity, and the most productive selected for future use. Both hybridomas and the monoclonal antibodies generated were then stored in liquid nitrogen.

The development of the hybridoma technique was a methodological mile-stone in biomedicine. It finally made possible the on-demand creation of identical, monoclonal, highly targeted immunoglobulins with preselected specificities, which could be provided in unlimited supplies. In 1984, Milstein and Köhler were awarded the Nobel Prize in Physiology or Medicine for discovering "the principle for production of monoclonal antibodies." They did not patent their method, which opened up the use of hybridoma technology to academic and pharmaceutical research worldwide.

Over the course of the following decade, hybridoma production was increasingly refined and expanded. Newer genetic engineering techniques replaced murine gene sequences with their human counterparts, resulting in chimeric (part mouse, part human) and eventually in near-fully humanized antibodies (approximately 95 percent human molecules). In 1986 British biochemist Greg Winter and his team developed humanized monoclonal antibodies using phage display, a technique in which bacteriophages connect proteins with their encoding genes. These innovations eliminated many adverse reactions caused by the immunogenicity of murine or chimeric antibodies. At the same time, easier—in Milstein's words, "à la carte"—production techniques provided the impetus for rapid marketing of useful antibodies. The same year, a first commercially approved monoclonal antibody was used to prevent kidney transplant rejection.

The advent of these "designer antibodies" opened up new conceptual avenues in understanding disease. In biomedical research, monoclonal antibodies became a quasi-limitless source of therapeutic and diagnostic agents. They are used for blood and tissue typing, and have enabled faster and more accurate clinical testing in many conditions. Diagnostic enzyme-linked immune-sorbent assays (ELISAs) identify specific infectious disease pathogens through mAb recognition of their unique antigenic features. In pregnancy tests, monoclonal antibodies bind to human chorionic gonadotropin (hCG) hormone made in the early stages of pregnancy. When tagged with radioactive isotopes in radioimmunoassays (RIAs), they scan for cancer cells and aid in early diagnosis.

Monoclonal antibodies have also become a major immunotherapeutic modality in various types of cancers, in autoimmune and infectious diseases, and in transplant and cardiovascular medicine. They can be aimed at almost any cellular or extracellular target to destroy malignant cells or prevent their growth by blocking specific receptors. They have led to advances such as recombinant interferon and insulin, and personalized drug therapies like Herceptin for breast cancer or Humira for rheumatoid arthritis. Today, there are approximately 30 mAbs approved for clinical use. Many more are undergoing clinical trial testing and are expected to revolutionize future disease therapies.

Bibliography and Suggested Readings

Buss, Nicholas, et al., "Monoclonal Antibody Therapeutics: History and Future," *Current Opinion in Pharmacology* October 2012, 12(5): 615–622.

Justin, K. H. Liu, "The History of Monoclonal Antibody Development—Progress, Remaining Challenges and Future Innovations," *Annals of Medicine and Surgery* December 2014, 3(4): 113–116.

Köhler, Georges, and Milstein, César, "Continuous Cultures of Fused Cells Secreting Antibody of Predefined Specificity," *Nature* 1975, 256: 495–497.

Marks, Lara, *The Lock and Key of Medicine: Monoclonal Antibodies and the Transformation of Healthcare*, New Haven: Yale University Press, 2015.

Siddiqui, Mahtab Z., "Monoclonal Antibodies as Diagnostics: An Appraisal," *Indian Journal of Pharmaceutical Sciences* 2010, 72(1): 12–17.

Waldmann, Herman, and Milstein, Celia, "The Antibody Problem and the Generation of Monoclonal Antibodies," in *Nobel Prizes That Changed Medicine,* ed. Gilbert Thompson, Singapore: World Scientific Publishing Co., 2011, pp. 197–215.

What Is Biotechnology?, http://www.whatisbiotechnology.org/home.

Vaccination

What	Administration of an antigenic substance to induce production of antibodies and protect the body against infectious disease; first used against smallpox.
Where	England
When	1796
By Whom	Edward Jenner (1749–1823)
Importance	Made possible control and prevention of infectious diseases; had a major impact on public health by reducing mortality and morbidity due to preventable infections; led to the eradication of smallpox; gave rise to the field of immunology.

Vaccination, the practice of administering a preventive substance to confer immunity against a specific disease, remains to this day one of the most extraordinary medical advances. First discovered in the 18th century to protect against epidemic smallpox, routine vaccination of large population groups has become an established practice and has contributed dramatically to improved global health.

The term vaccination is derived from the word *vaccinia*, after the Latin *vacca*, cow. Coined by English physician Edward Jenner, it denoted a disease known as cowpox (*variola vaccina*), a viral infection of cows. The cowpox virus, *vaccinia*, is closely related to the *variola* virus, the causative agent of the highly infectious and often fatal smallpox. Smallpox, an ancient disease, sickened and killed millions of people over the centuries. The devastating smallpox epidemics of the early modern era had mortality rates ranging from 30 percent to as high as 90 percent. The characteristic pustular rash of smallpox produced deeply pitted scars that often left survivors permanently disfigured; some were blinded due to corneal scarring. Rich and poor were equally affected. In 17th- and 18th-century Europe, smallpox had supplanted plague as the most feared pestilence. There were also frequent outbreaks in the American colonies where smallpox would decimate indigenous populations.

It was generally believed—even though microbial organisms as disease agents were yet to be discovered—that smallpox was contagious and that its victims must be isolated. Because there was no effective treatment, medical efforts focused on preventing outbreaks and protecting against the disease. It was known that smallpox survivors were resistant to future outbreaks and that healthy individuals could be made immune by exposure to the pus of infected persons. Early techniques, documented in 17th-century China and India, entailed the breathing in of powdered scabs from smallpox victims. Another process known as "variolation" or "inoculation" was to instill the thick fluid matter contained in fresh smallpox pustules into the arms or legs of a healthy, nonimmune person by means of a lancet. People so inoculated usually suffered only a mild illness, and their risk of serious disease or death was much less. In the early 1700s, the practice of variolation spread to England, largely through the advocacy of Lady Mary Wortley Montague, wife of the British ambassador to Turkey. A victim of smallpox herself, she had the procedure successfully performed on both her children. Variolation, although controversial and not without risks, was gradually adopted. By 1755, the Royal College of Physicians unanimously judged it to be "of the utmost benefit to mankind," making it an accepted medical practice.

But the method devised by British physician Edward Jenner was equally effective and much safer than variolation. Jenner's procedure consisted of inoculating infectious cowpox material. A bovine form of smallpox, cowpox manifested itself by ulcers on cows' udders; when transmitted to humans, it mostly caused localized lesions on the hands where skin cracks or abrasions allowed entry of the virus. Importantly, however, such exposures also appeared to create immunity to smallpox. Indeed, it was widely observed among rural people that dairymaids, who milked the cows, were somehow shielded from smallpox. Jenner reportedly overheard a dairymaid's claim that because she had had cowpox, she would be immune to smallpox.

In 1796, during an outbreak of cowpox among local milkmaids at a Gloucestershire farm, he extracted some fluid from Sarah Nelmes, a young milkmaid infected with cowpox, and with this fluid inoculated a small boy. The boy, eight-year-old James Phipps, suffered only a mild reaction and recovered fully. The following summer Jenner subjected the boy to variolation, inoculating him with true smallpox. Phipps remained healthy, exhibited no signs of smallpox, and thus demonstrated the preventive effect of cowpox vaccination. Jenner published his findings in 1798 in a landmark monograph entitled *"Inquiry into the Causes and Effects of the Variolae Vaccinae"* where he described a total of 23 cases. His conclusions were that "the Cow Pox protects the human constitution from the infection of the Small Pox . . ."

Jenner had effectively developed the first viral vaccine against smallpox. He had successfully tested "an antidote . . . capable of extirpating from the earth a disease which is every hour devouring its victims; a disease that has ever been considered as the severest scourge of the human race!" Within a decade, his technique had spread around the globe. Over the course of the 19th century, in spite of continued controversy, Jennerian vaccination became compulsory in most European countries and in Canada. In 1840, the British Parliament outlawed variolation. Disease incidence declined steadily until 1977 when the last case of natural smallpox was recorded in Somalia. Two years later the World Health Organization (WHO) formally declared smallpox dead, a goal achieved through its global vaccination effort. Because smallpox only infects humans, vaccination eradicated the disease by eliminating its natural reservoir.

Letter from Thomas Jefferson, third president of the United States (1801–1809) to Edward Jenner:

To Dr. Edward Jenner   Monticello, May 14, 1806

SIR,

I have received a copy of the evidence at large respecting the discovery of the vaccine inoculation which you have been pleased to send me, and for which I return you my thanks. Having been among the early converts, in this part of the globe, to its efficiency, I took an early part in recommending it to my countrymen. I avail myself of this occasion of rendering you a portion of the tribute of gratitude due to you from the whole human family. Medicine has never before produced any single improvement of such utility. Harvey's discovery of the circulation of the blood was a beautiful addition to our knowledge of the animal economy, but on a review of the practice of medicine before and since that epoch, I do not see any great amelioration which has been derived from that discovery.

You have erased from the calendar of human afflictions one of its greatest. Yours is the comfortable reflection that mankind can never forget that you have lived. Future nations will know by history only that the loathsome small-pox has existed and by you has been extirpated.

Accept my fervent wishes for your health and happiness and assurances of the greatest respect and consideration.

Thomas Jefferson

Source: *Public Health Reports*, volume 23, part 1, January 31, 1908.

Jenner's technique of substituting a weaker infectious agent to induce immunity eventually evolved into modern-day vaccination, the routine preventive use of innocuous forms of the actual disease agent. In the 19th century Louis Pasteur was the first to develop killed vaccines against rabies and anthrax by manipulating the infectious agents so as to render them less virulent; he adopted the term *vaccine* in honor of Jenner's discovery. Over the course of the two centuries that followed Jenner's groundbreaking work, vaccination would be extended to a number of other infectious diseases, including diphtheria, hepatitis A and B, measles, tetanus, and poliomyelitis. Nine vaccine-preventable infections for which childhood vaccination was universally recommended before 1990 have seen dramatic declines in mortality and morbidity rates: 100 percent for smallpox, and nearly 100 percent for the others.

Today's vaccines consist of killed, inactivated, or attenuated (weakened) bacteria or virus to stimulate antibody production. The *vaccinia* virus used in modern vaccines is a hybrid virus, which probably evolved from inadvertent contamination of cowpox cultures with smallpox in the early years of vaccination; it still confers immunity to smallpox.

Bibliography and Suggested Readings

Bazin, Hervé, *The Eradication of Small Pox*, New York: Academic Press, 2000.

Centers for Disease Control and Prevention, "Impact of Vaccines Universally Recommended for Children," *Morbidity and Mortality Weekly Report*, April 2, 1999, 48(12): 243–248.

Gaynes, Robert P., *Germ Theory: Medical Pioneers in Infectious Diseases*, Washington, DC: ASM Press, 2011.

Jenner, Edward, *An Inquiry into the Causes and Effects of the Variolae Vaccinae*, 1798, http://www.gutenberg.org/ebooks/29414.

McNeil, William H., *Plagues and Peoples*, New York: Anchor Publications, 1976.

Vitamins

What	Organic compounds recognized to be essential nutrients necessary for normal growth and metabolism.
Where	Netherlands; United Kingdom; Hungary; United States; Germany
When	1890 to 1920s
By Whom	Christiaan Eijkman (1858–1930); Sir Frederick Gowland Hopkins (1861–1947); Casimir Funk (1884–1967); Joseph Goldberger (1874–1929); many others
Importance	Made possible prevention and treatment of deficiency diseases; helped establish modern nutritional science.

Vitamins are organic compounds essential for life. All have highly specific functions required for health and normal development. Some have an enzymatic or antioxidant action, aiding to regulate metabolic growth processes or to store or release energy; others are chemically related to steroid molecules and act as hormones. Vitamins are often classified according to their solubility, either in fat or in water. Water-soluble vitamins are absorbed by the gut and carried by the bloodstream to the tissues where in combination with proteins they form active enzymes catalyzing various metabolic processes. When their intake exceeds the body's requirements, the excess is excreted in the urine. Fat-soluble vitamins are absorbed within small fat globules, transported in the lymphatic system, and primarily stored in the liver and in fatty tissue.

Thirteen compounds are generally recognized as vitamins, four fat-soluble, nine water-soluble. Until their chemical composition was known, they were categorized alphabetically as vitamins A, B, C, D, etc., mostly in order of their discovery, except for the large collection of compounds known as B complex vitamins. The coagulation factor vitamin K, indispensable for blood clotting, takes its name from the German term, "Koagulation."

The existence of special dietary factors had long been suspected. When 19th-century advances in biochemistry ushered in scientific food studies, most focused on protein, fats, and carbohydrates and their conversion into energy for metabolic needs. It was known that inadequate intake of food stuffs resulted in starvation and death. Yet, early observations also indicated that the body had a need for nutrients other than protein, fat, and sugar, but the connection between nutrition and specific disorders had not been established. By the late 1800s, it became clear that there were added requirements for a healthful diet and that various pathological conditions were likely due to deficiency states rather than to toxic disease factors.

Between 1900 and 1922, several diseases were linked to a deficit of specific substances not yet chemically identified: growth retardation, xerophthalmia (pathological dryness of cornea and conjunctiva) and poor night vision (linked to lack of vitamin A), beriberi (vitamin B_1), scurvy (vitamin C), rickets (vitamin D), and pellagra (vitamin B_3). These discoveries radically altered contemporary scientific and pathophysiological views and redirected the course of nutritional research.

Associated with diet from an early stage was beriberi (from the Sinhalese, "very weak"), a peripheral nerve disease first encountered by 19th-century European colonialists in Dutch Indonesia and Malaysia. Beriberi had become common in Southeast Asia ever since rice was produced with new steam-operated rice mills, which polished the grains (and removed B_1 vitamins). Symptoms of beriberi were weakness, loss of sensation in the limbs, swelling, difficulty breathing, and ultimately death through heart failure. Found in prisons and other institutional settings, the condition appeared to be related to consumption of milled or polished "white" rice, rather than to raw, unprocessed "brown" rice. Most physicians assumed a microbial basis for the disease, but in 1890 Dutch medical officer Christiaan Eijkman showed that chickens fed on a diet of soldiers' leftover white rice developed a characteristic leg weakness; they were cured when the rice husk millings were returned to their feed. Eijkman's colleague Gerrit Grijns correctly concluded that the disease was not due to a toxic level of starch, but that rice polishings must contain a substance essential to prevent peripheral nerve injury.

In 1906, English biochemist Frederick Gowland Hopkins confirmed this view. Hopkins's experiments with rats showed that a diet consisting only of pure proteins, carbohydrates, fats, minerals, and water failed to support growth; only animals fed supplementary milk grew normally. He concluded that small amounts of certain "accessory food factors" as yet unidentified were essential for growth. In 1912, Lister Institute scientist Casimir Funk tried to isolate the active anti-beriberi factor; he suggested that rice husks contained a vital amine (compound derived from ammonia), or "vitamine," and that a number of conditions derived from dietary lack of these essential compounds. Funk's term for these "accessory factors" was eventually reduced to *vitamin*, when it became clear that not all vitamins were amines.

In 1913, Yale University researchers Osborne and Mendel showed that butter contained an essential growth factor, determined to be fat-soluble vitamin A. A similar factor was found in egg yolk and cod liver oil. The chemical structure

The Pellagra "Germ"

Pellagra, often mistaken for leprosy, was known as the disease of the three D's—dermatitis, diarrhea, and dementia. In the early 1900s it reached epidemic proportions in prisons and orphanages of the U.S. South. A 1914 congressional commission concluded that pellagra was "in all probability a specific infectious disease communicable . . . by means at present unknown." The U.S. Public Health Service appointed one of its officers, Dr. Joseph Goldberger, to investigate. Goldberger's observations quickly convinced him that the disease could not be contagious. Indeed, those who attended the pellagrins were never infected; in mental hospitals, prisons, and orphanages, only inmates contracted pellagra, but staff never did.

Instead, diet seemed to be a key factor. Goldberger confirmed this theory by adding a daily egg, two glasses of milk, and a serving of meat to the corn-based diet of a Mississippi orphanage where 60 percent of children had pellagra. A few months later there was not one case! Goldberger corroborated his findings with an experiment on 12 healthy prisoners, who were offered unconditional pardons in exchange for a six-month corn-based diet. Afterward, Goldberger wrote to his wife that he had "really and truly produced pellagra in great big and vigorous men by just feeding them improperly."

Nevertheless, many remained unconvinced. Some even accused Goldberger of having falsified his results. Goldberger ultimately subjected himself to a series of experiments to prove that pellagra was not contagious. Years later, Mary Goldberger remembered how her late husband and his assistant wiped noses and mouths of pellagra patients with cotton swabs, which they then immediately rubbed over their own mucosa and nasopharynx. They even swallowed capsules containing "the most nauseating diabolical concoctions [made up of . . . blood, feces, and urine of pellagra patients]." Mary herself was injected with the blood of a woman dying of pellagra. Neither Goldberger nor his more than 20 volunteers ever developed any symptoms of pellagra.

We know today that pellagra is a deficiency disease caused by lack of vitamin B_3, niacin. Goldberger himself did not identify the vitamin, but his groundbreaking work contributed to laying the foundation for modern nutritional science.

of vitamin A was established in 1933, and it was synthesized in 1947. Cow's milk, wheat and rice bran, and yeast contained another water-soluble growth factor, named vitamin B; necessary to prevent beriberi, it was synthesized in 1936.

At the same time, Leonard Findlay in Glasgow, Edward Mellanby in London, and Elmer McCollum at Johns Hopkins focused on elucidating the cause of rickets, widespread among young children in industrial cities on both sides of the Atlantic. Rickets, a weakening and softening of bones when mineralization is defective, could be cured by cod liver oil, which in 1922 was found to contain the "anti-rachitic factor": vitamin D. Essential to calcium metabolism and bone formation, active vitamin D is synthesized by the body upon exposure to sunlight. Milk enriched with vitamin D, first introduced in 1933, proved very effective in combating the disease. The same year, another fat-soluble factor necessary for normal reproduction was identified as vitamin E.

Progress was also made in the investigation of scurvy, a disease due to deficiency of vitamin C, which is essential to human collagen synthesis. Characterized by weakness, joint pains, loose teeth, subcutaneous hemorrhages, poor wound healing, and ultimate death if untreated, the condition had been described in Hippocratic times. It had long been known that sailors on long voyages would develop scurvy if their diet lacked fruit or green vegetables. Empiric treatments were recorded as early as the 1500s; French explorer Jacques Cartier in 1535 used a native decoction of pine needles (rich in vitamin C) to cure his crew afflicted with scurvy. As early as 1830 a London lecturer taught that scurvy was a "chemical disease," caused by the lack of a "necessary thing" contained in fresh food. Nineteenth-century German pathologist August Hirsch had found potatoes to be antiscorbutic, and London hospital doctors treated scurvy in children with diets of milk, meat, potatoes, and citrus juice.

In 1907, Norwegian scientists studying dietary factors in beriberi accidentally reproduced scurvy in guinea pigs, paving the way for a series of investigations at the London Lister Institute that ultimately led to the isolation of the antiscorbutic factor. By 1919, it was recognized as an essential nutrient, and in 1932 Hungarian scientist Albert Szent-Györgyi first synthesized vitamin C in his laboratory. Called ascorbic acid, the substance was easily destroyed by heat and by contact with metal—which explained the long-ago therapeutic failure of sea captain James Lind's evaporated lime juice.

In an era of new microbiological theories of disease these studies contributed to establishing a new paradigm, the notion that disease could arise from a *lack* of vital substances rather than from a *presence* of a germ or toxin. This concept became central to the development of modern nutritional science.

The Nobel Prize Committee acknowledged, albeit with some delay, the critical importance of work involving nutrition. Starting in 1929, at least 10 awards recognized specific research involving the discovery of vitamins:

Nobel Prize in Physiology or Medicine

1929   Christiaan Eijkman "for his discovery of the antineuritic vitamin" (vitamin B_1); Sir Frederick Gowland Hopkins "for his discovery of the growth-stimulating vitamins"

1934   George Hoyt Whipple, George Richards Minot, and William Parry Murphy, "for their discoveries concerning liver therapy in cases of anemia" (vitamin B_{12})

1937   Albert von Szent-Györgyi Nagyrápolt "for his discoveries in connection with the biological combustion processes, with special reference to vitamin C . . ."

1943   Henrik Carl Peter Dam "for his discovery of vitamin K" and Edward Adelbert Doisy "for his discovery of the chemical nature of vitamin K"

Nobel Prize in Chemistry

1928   Adolf Otto Reinhold Windaus "for the services rendered through his research into the constitution of the sterols and their connection with the vitamins" (vitamin D)

1937   Walter Norman Haworth "for his investigations on carbohydrates and vitamin C" and Paul Karrer "for his investigations on carotenoids, flavins and vitamins A and B_2"

1938   Richard Kuhn "for his work on carotenoids and vitamins" (vitamins B_2 and B_6)

1964   Dorothy Crowfoot Hodgkin "for her determinations by X-ray techniques of the structures of important biochemical substances" (vitamin B_{12})

Today, most physiological functions of vitamins and their molecular structures have been determined. Vitamins can be manufactured synthetically and are used in the food industry, where large quantities are added to animal feed. There is no uniform agreement about vitamin requirements for a healthy human diet. It is generally thought that a balanced diet supplies all the vitamins needed for health maintenance, but this does not always hold true. Malnutrition and vitamin deficiencies are found both in poor and in affluent societies, and are more common in the elderly, in pregnant women, and in children; they may be a result of low intake, increased requirements, or impaired absorption.

Cultural, political, and economic factors can significantly affect vitamin intake and lead to endemic deficiencies and disease.

Starting in 1936, after the synthesis of vitamins C and B_2, vitamin supplements became ever more popular, in part based on the belief that adding to a minimum required intake would lead to better health and longer life. In the United States, the production of vitamins and dietary supplements has become a multibillion-dollar industry. Manufacturers must register their facilities with the Food and Drug Administration (FDA), but are not required to get FDA approval before producing or selling dietary supplements.

Bibliography and Suggested Readings

Apple, Rima D., *Vitamania: Vitamins in American Culture, New Brunswick:* Rutgers University Press, 1996.

Carpenter, Kenneth J., "Nutritional Chemistry," in *The Cambridge World History of Human Disease*, ed. Kenneth F. Kiple, Cambridge: Cambridge University Press, 1993: 140–147.

Carpenter, Kenneth J., *The History of Scurvy and Vitamin C,* Cambridge: Cambridge University Press, 1986.

Carpenter, Kenneth J., *Beriberi, White Rice, and Vitamin B: A Disease, a Cause, and a Cure.* Berkeley: University of California Press, 2000.

Carpenter, Kenneth J., "The Nobel Prize and the Discovery of Vitamins," 2004, http://www.nobelprize.org/nobel_prizes/themes/medicine/carpenter.

Coley, Nicola, "Vitamins," in *Encyclopedia of 20th Century Technology,* eds. Colin A. Hempstead, et al., Vol. 2, London: Routledge, 2005.

Coulston, Ann M., "Vitamins," in *Encyclopedia of Food and Culture*, ed. Solomon H. Katz, Vol. 3. New York: Charles Scribner's Sons, 2003, pp. 497–503.

Goldberger, Mary F., "Dr. Joseph Goldberger: His Wife's Recollections," in *Essays on History of Nutrition and Dietetics*, compiled by Beeuwkes, Adelia, et al., Chicago: The American Dietetic Association, 1967, pp. 103–106.

Herrmann, W., and Obeid, R., eds., *Vitamins in the Prevention of Human Diseases*, Berlin: Walter de Gruyter, 2011.

McDowell, Lee, *Vitamin History: The Early Years, Sarasota:* University of Florida, 2013.

Brief Timeline of Medical Innovations

ca. 100 A.D.—The earliest **hospitals** appear throughout the Roman Empire. They were infirmaries (*valetudinaria*) for wounded soldiers and also functioned as storehouses for supplies.

ca. 1280—The earliest wearable **eyeglasses** are invented in Italy. Used by scholars and clerics, they are held in front of the eyes with a metal handle or balanced on the nose. Prior to this "reading stones"—hemispherical lenses made of glass or crystal—were laid over the text for magnification.

1546—In his treatise *De Contagione,* Italian scientist Girolamo Fracastoro sets forth a **germ theory of disease** stating that epidemic diseases are transmitted by tiny, invisible particles, or "seeds."

1561—Ambroise Paré's *Universal Surgery* revolutionizes the traditional treatment of wounds. Instead of boiling oil and cautery, Paré advocates gentle **cleansing of wounds** and ligatures to control hemorrhage.

1590—Dutch spectacle maker Janssen introduces the earliest compound **microscope**. Instead of a single-lens magnifying glass, it consists of drawtubes for focusing, with a bi-convex eyepiece and a plano-convex objective lens.

1592—Galileo constructs the first rudimentary **thermometer**.

1612—Santorio adds a numerical scale to Galileo's early "thermoscope" to measure abnormal body temperatures.

1628—William Harvey publishes the first explanation of the **continuous circulation of the blood** showing that it is pumped within the body in a closed system. His work underpins modern-day understanding of blood circulation.

1630—Jesuit missionaries in Peru begin exporting to Europe the bark of the cinchona tree, which "produced miraculous results" in treating certain febrile illnesses. In Europe, the powdered "fever" or "Jesuit's" bark revolutionizes traditional concepts of disease as imbalance of the humors. **Cinchona bark** acted quickly and specifically on the fever caused by malaria and was the main antimalarial agent until 1820 when it was found to contain **quinine**.

1661—Italian scientist Marcello Malpighi, an expert microscopist, discovers the existence of **capillaries** and confirms the connection between arteries and veins postulated by Harvey.

1665—Dutch scientist Christiaan Huygens proposes a fixed **thermometric scale** using the freezing and boiling points of water. Designated as 0 and 100 degrees, respectively, they become the origin of the centigrade system.

1674—Antony van Leeuwenhoek, a Dutch cloth merchant, builds the first high-power single-lens "**microscope**." He describes molds, yeasts, blood and sperm cells, bee stings, and the stripes of striated muscle fibers. He also discovers live bacteria in dental plaque, "animalcules . . . in such enormous numbers, that all the spittle . . . seemed to be alive."

1717—Daniel **Fahrenheit** introduces smaller increments as well as **mercury**, which expands and contracts more rapidly than water, into his **thermometer**.

ca. 1720—Hermann Boerhaave and his students bring **thermometry** into clinical practice. They report daily cyclical temperature changes in healthy patients and study the relationship between temperature and pulse.

ca. 1728—The introduction of the previously secret **Chamberlen obstetrical forceps** is a critical advance and stimulates development of surgical obstetrics. The instrument aids successful extraction of a live child from the vaginal canal during difficult births.

1733—English clergyman Stephen Hales publishes his experiments on the dynamics of blood circulation and **blood pressure** measures in several animals. His manometer is a forerunner of modern-day **sphygmomanometers**.

1742—Swedish astronomer Anders **Celsius** reintroduces the centigrade system and develops an improved **thermometer**.

1747—The experiments of Scottish naval surgeon James Lind establish that **citrus** fruits are superior to all other remedies in the treatment of **scurvy**.

1761—Vienna physician Leopold Auenbrugger introduces **diagnostic percussion**, during which the examiner taps parts of the patient's body with his fingers while listening closely to the acoustic quality of the elicited sounds. Percussion becomes an important diagnostic technique before the days of medical imaging, helping to assess abnormal densities in underlying tissues.

1763—In a letter to the Royal Society, English clergyman and scholar Edmund Stone first reports the beneficial effects of **willow bark** in relieving fever and pain. Chewing of salicin-containing willow bark, from which is derived the future **aspirin (salicylic acid)**, was already advised in Hippocratic times for reducing fever and inflammation.

1774–1794—Joseph Priestley and Antoine Lavoisier discover **oxygen** and the role of oxygen in combustion, critical to understanding the physiology of respiration and the process of oxidation in living cells.

1780s—Bologna scientist Luigi Galvani hypothesizes that animal tissues have inherent electrical properties responsible for physiological processes such as nerve conduction and muscle contraction. His observations on the excitability of frog muscle fibers lay the foundation for **electrophysiology**.

1785—Physician and botanist William Withering publishes a first systematic description of the clinical effects of foxglove, *Digitalis purpurea*, used in folk medicine for treating dropsy, the swelling of the body, and difficult breathing caused by severe heart failure. **Digitalis**, which improves myocardial contractility, was employed long before its chemical structure and mechanism of action were determined.

1798—Edward Jenner reports on the effectiveness of **vaccination** in protecting against smallpox by inoculating people with the fluid of cowpox (*vaccinia*) sores. The previous technique, variolation (from *variola*, smallpox) where serous fluid from human smallpox is inoculated so as to produce a mild case of disease, had limited success and could be lethal.

1806—Philipp Bozzini publishes his "invention for viewing internal parts and diseases." This early **endoscopic instrument** helped localize bladder stones and, after childbirth, identify sources of vaginal bleeding.

1806 and 1817—German apprentice pharmacist Friedrich Sertürner succeeds in extracting **morphine** from crude opium. Morphine becomes one of the most important drug discoveries of the 19th century. Initially used only orally, its use spreads after the development of the hypodermic syringe in the 1850s.

1816—René Laënnec invents the **stethoscope** to aid in listening to patients' chest sounds. Until then, heart and lung sounds were examined by pressing one's ear against the patient's chest. By 1850 Laënnec's monaural wooden cylinder is developed into a device with two earpieces and becomes the standard clinical tool still in use today.

1820—French chemists Joseph Caventou and Pierre Pelletier isolate **quinine**, the active ingredient of cinchona bark. Purified quinine replaces the bark and remains the only effective antimalarial until the mid-20th century.

1835—Pierre Charles Louis publishes his classic study on the efficacy of standard treatments for pneumonia, demonstrating that bloodletting does more harm than good. His "numerical method" becomes a major force in the development of **clinical trials** and scientific evaluation for all therapies.

1842—Georgia physician Crawford Long performs the first surgical operation using **ether** anesthesia to remove two small tumors from the neck of a patient.

1844–1846—Connecticut dentist Horace Wells tries **nitrous oxide** ("laughing gas") as an anesthetic while having one of his own teeth removed. The following year, in Boston, a failed demonstration to medical students ends in his public embarrassment. In 1846, Wells's former partner William T. G. Morton and surgeon John Collins Warren perform the first successful public trial of inhaled **ether anesthesia**. News quickly spreads around the world. The Massachusetts General Hospital surgical theater has been preserved in memory of the event as the *Ether Dome*.

1847—Scottish obstetrician James Young Simpson champions the anesthetic properties of **chloroform** for the relief of labor pains in the face of much opposition. The clergy denounces him for disregarding scriptural admonition (that women shall bring forth children "in sorrow"). John Snow, whose research on inhaled anesthetics contributes to developing the new discipline of **anesthesia,** famously used chloroform when attending Queen Victoria at the birth of her eighth child in 1853.

1845–1849—Alabama physician James Marion Sims perfects surgical repair of vesicovaginal fistula, a severe complication of childbirth where tearing of the tissue between the woman's vagina and bladder results in fistulous tracts with continuous, uncontrollable leakage of urine. Sims devises a special **speculum** to aid in his operation. His experimenting on vulnerable black slave women has led to ongoing ethical debate.

1847—Ignaz Semmelweis pioneers **antisepsis** in maternity wards and dramatically reduces the incidence of the frequently fatal childbed fever.

1851—German physicist-physician Hermann von Helmholtz devises the first **ophthalmoscope** making the inner eye visible to an examiner. His instrument consists of a concave mirror with a central hole, shining light into the pupil and enabling the viewer to see the reflection of the retina.

1853—The **hypodermic syringe** is developed for clinical use. Syringe barrels are initially made of metal but are soon made of glass to aid in dosing injected medicines.

1854—English physician John Snow identifies the public water pump on Broad Street as the source of a cholera outbreak in London's Soho district that killed more than 600 people. By carefully tracking and mapping cases of disease victims, he establishes the link between cholera and use of the contaminated well; after he convinces officials to remove the pump's handle (making it impossible to draw water), the epidemic subsides. Years before Pasteur's germ theory and later Koch's discovery of the cholera "poison," Snow's pioneering investigations lay the groundwork for the future field of **epidemiology** and **health geography**; modern-day epidemiological research still uses Snow's innovative methods to trace the causes of many diseases. Cholera remains an ongoing **public health** concern in areas of the world without adequate sanitation of water supplies.

1859—Louis Pasteur proves the existence of invisible microorganisms in the air and proposes that they are responsible for **contagion**. His subsequent research and that of Robert Koch establish proof for the **germ theory of disease**, the single most significant medical advance of the 19th century.

1862—After an accidental discovery of crystals in blood samples, German physician Felix Hoppe-Seyler coins the word **hemoglobin** for the "colorant substance of blood" and shows how it binds oxygen in red blood cells.

1863–1864—Swiss businessman Jean Henri Dunant founds the **International Red Cross**. A witness to the horrific bloodshed and suffering of the 1859 battle of Solferino, Dunant calls for an international relief organization to care for the sick and wounded on the battlefield, no matter which side they belong to. In the 1864 Geneva Convention, 12 signatory nations lay down treatment guidelines for all wounded combatants and guarantee neutrality and protection to medical and sanitary personnel. Dunant is awarded the first Nobel Peace Prize in 1901 for his humanitarian work.

1865—Inspired by Pasteur's research, Joseph Lister starts applying **antiseptic principles** to his surgical practice and in 1867 reports that sterilization with carbolic acid significantly reduces postoperative infections. Lister's insistence on sanitary conditions and strict cleanliness during operations transforms surgical practice.

1867–1868—British physician Thomas Albutt designs the first portable thermometer, replacing a long cumbersome instrument with a 6-inch pocket-size model. Meanwhile, German Carl Wunderlich analyzes temperature variations in thousands of patients showing that fever is not a disease, but an important symptom; he helps popularize the **clinical thermometer**.

1880s—Sterile **intracapsular cataract extractions** under topical anesthesia replace the traditional cataract "couching" technique.

1881—Louis Pasteur discovers that growing anthrax bacilli in specific conditions renders them harmless yet preserves their capacity to produce resistance when injected. His findings lead to the first attenuated **anthrax vaccine** and establish that attenuated cultures of a microbe protect against disease caused by the same microbe, a fundamental **principle of immunity**. In 1885, Pasteur and collaborator Émile Roux develop a first **rabies vaccine** based on the same principle and demonstrate its efficacy in Joseph Meister, a nine-year-old boy who had been attacked by a rabid dog.

1882—Robert Koch identifies *Mycobacterium tuberculosis*, the bacillus responsible for **tuberculosis**, then a leading cause of death.

1883—Koch isolates the bacterium that causes **cholera**, an acute diarrheal disease due to contaminated food or drink.

1888—Swiss physician Eugen Fick develops the first glass **contact lenses**. His lenses cover the entire eye, not just the cornea, but they are too thick to be worn all day.

1890—Emile Roux and Alexandre Yersin show that diphtheria produces a poisonous toxin in the bloodstream. Emil von Behring develops an effective **diphtheria antitoxin** by injecting increasing doses of toxin into animals to render them immune. Serum containing protective antibodies is used to treat others exposed to the disease, providing **"passive" immunization**. The following year Behring's **serum therapy**—diphtheria antitoxin from convalescent serum—is used successfully to treat infected children.

1895—Wilhelm Röntgen discovers a new type of electromagnetic wave that he calls **X-ray**. The new rays can penetrate the human body and make visible its internal structures on a photographic plate without surgery.

1895—**Iodine** is discovered in the thyroid gland. The trace element is necessary for the production of thyroid hormone, essential for normal growth and metabolism.

1896—Scipione Riva-Rocci introduces his method for measuring blood pressure by compressing the brachial artery with an inflatable band. His new device is the prototypical modern **sphygmomanometer**.

1897—Felix Hoffmann purifies the active ingredient of willow bark, salicin or **salicylic acid**. The new drug is shown to have excellent anti-inflammatory and analgesic properties, and in 1899 is registered by manufacturer Bayer as *Aspirin*.

1897—Giovanni Battista Grassi and Ronald Ross independently demonstrate the link between human **malaria** and the *Plasmodium* parasite through infected *Anopheles* mosquitoes, which transmit the disease.

1900—Karl Landsteiner observes that mixing blood of some people with that of others causes clumping and destruction of blood cells. His studies lead to the discovery of the major **human blood groups, A, B, O,** and later **AB,** and to the achievement of safe blood transfusions.

1900—Austrian physician Sigmund Freud begins developing the conceptual framework for **psychoanalysis**, revolutionizing early 20th-century psychiatry. He emphasizes the role of childhood experiences, internal psychological conflict, and the subconscious in the development of mental life and psychopathology. While Freud's theories of human behavior remain influential in certain quarters, current research in neurophysiology, psychopharmacology, and genetics centers on the physical structure of the brain and on the biochemical and biomolecular substrates of psychological processes and mental illness.

1901—Ivan **Pavlov**, a distinguished Russian physiologist, develops his theory of **learning and conditioning**, which explores and highlights connections between physiology and behavior, and becomes a lasting influence in neurophysiology and behaviorism. Pavlov is awarded a Nobel Prize in 1904 for his work on the physiology of digestion.

1901—German psychiatrist Alois Alzheimer identifies the first case of what has become known as **Alzheimer's disease**, a neurodegenerative form of dementia.

1902—Alexis Carrel develops a highly effective **suturing method** for connecting blood vessels end to end; his **anastomosis** technique becomes indispensable in later organ transplantation.

1903—Willem Einthoven invents the **electrocardiograph (ECG or EKG)**, which measures the electrical activity of the heart and translates it into defined visual tracings that reflect normal and abnormal myocardial conduction. Electrocardiographic diagnosis has become a cornerstone of clinical cardiology.

1906—Frederick Hopkins's experiments with rats show that certain "accessory food factors" are essential for normal growth and development. Their lack causes **nutritional deficiency** diseases such as rickets or scurvy. In 1912 Casimir Funk coins the term "vital amine," later contracted to **vitamin**.

1906—August von Wassermann devises a specific blood test for syphilis antibodies based on the complement fixation reaction. The **Wassermann test** was the first to make possible diagnostic screening for the disease.

1907—Clemens von Pirquet and Béla Schick study hypersensitivity reactions, coining the word **allergy**, from the Greek "allos," other, and "ergon," action. Building on their work, Charles Mantoux develops the **Mantoux test**, also known as **PPD** (purified protein derivative) tuberculin, an extract of *M. tuberculosis*. The test is used worldwide as a major screening tool for tuberculosis.

1908—Karl Landsteiner and Erwin Popper are the first to identify the causative agent of **polio** as a **virus**.

1908—Victor Horsley and Robert Clarke at University College London invent the **stereotactic method** for minimally invasive surgery. The Horsley-Clarke apparatus uses spatial coordinates to guide surgical approach of small, poorly accessible internal structures.

1909—German physician Richard Richter reports insertion of the first **intrauterine device (IUD)**, a ring made of silkworm gut and two ends left protruding from the cervical opening for removal. The development of safe, effective IUDs in the 1960s has led to making this an increasingly popular method of long-acting and reversible contraception.

1909—Paul Ehrlich and his team synthesize the first modern chemotherapeutic antibiotic agents: arsphenamine, a toxic arsenical compound effective in treating syphilis, marketed as **Salvarsan** in 1910, and neoarsphenamine (Neo-Salvarsan), an improved form developed in 1914. Ehrlich's "magic bullets" transform the treatment of syphilis.

1910—Hans Christian Jacobaeus, a Swedish internist, performs the first percutaneous diagnostic **laparoscopies** on human patients. Today, minimally invasive laparoscopic techniques are used for numerous surgical procedures; the most common is cholecystectomy.

1915—Joseph Goldberger's experimental studies on healthy prison volunteers demonstrate the nutritional basis for **pellagra**, a disease caused by **niacin (vitamin B$_3$)** deficiency; niacin, or nicotinic acid, was identified in 1937 by University of Wisconsin biochemist Conrad Elvehjem.

1916–1918—**Heparin** (from the Greek "hepar," liver) is isolated from canine liver cells and shown to have anticoagulant properties. Naturally occurring in many animal tissues, especially liver, muscle, and lung, the substance is first tested in human trials in 1937. By the late 1940s a method is developed to produce large quantities of purified heparin for safe medical use. Heparin has many important indications, including prevention of postoperative thrombosis and embolism.

1920—Johnson & Johnson employee Earle Dickson invents the **Band-Aid** by affixing a strip of gauze to the center of a piece of adhesive tape and covering it with stiff protective fabric. His design becomes the famous trademarked adhesive bandage used worldwide to protect minor wounds.

1921—Frederick Banting and Charles Best isolate **insulin**, the pancreatic hormone essential for normal carbohydrate metabolism. Its absence or deficiency causes diabetes.

1921—Elmer McCollum and Edward Mellanby discover the antirachitic factor **vitamin D**. Deficiency results in rickets or osteomalacia, both conditions characterized by soft, weakened bones due to inadequate calcium absorption.

1922—Gaston Ramon develops the first safe and effective **diphtheria toxoid** by detoxifying the previously used toxin-antitoxin preparation with formaldehyde.

1922–1924—The Swiss Federation and the United States institute systematic **iodine supplementation of table salt** in areas where natural iodine is deficient. The programs result in marked reduction of endemic hypothyroid goiter.

1924–1928—Over 100,000 infants are vaccinated against tuberculosis (TB) with **BCG (Bacille Calmette-Guérin) vaccine**, the only vaccine for the prevention of TB. It is still in widespread use. Prepared from live attenuated strains, its efficacy has been controversial and there exists to date no global vaccination policy.

1926—American scientists discover that pernicious anemia, a fatal disease, is treatable with large amounts of dietary liver. The missing factor is later identified as **vitamin B$_{12}$**.

1928—The first **artificial respirator** is built at Harvard to treat polio victims. Using two vacuum cleaners, this "**iron lung**" expands and compresses patients' paralyzed chests by raising and lowering pressures within a steel enclosure.

1928—Returning to his lab after a short holiday, Alexander Fleming discovers the antimicrobial action of a mold and eventually concludes the substance might have therapeutic value. He names it **penicillin**.

1929—Trying to find a way to inject emergency medication directly into the heart, Werner Forssmann carries out the first **cardiac catheterization** on himself by pushing a ureteric catheter through a vein in his left arm into his right cardiac atrium. His innovative experiment proves essential to the future treatment of heart disease.

1929—Hans Berger publishes his technique for tracking the brain's electrical impulses from the surface of the head. He records the first human **electroencephalogram, or EEG**, in 1924.

1930s—French radiologist Henri Coutard pioneers a fractionated dosing process for therapeutic X-rays to reduce the hazardous effects of radiation exposure on healthy tissues. His intermittent low-dose delivery system carried out over several weeks becomes the basis for modern **cancer radiotherapy**, making possible the cure of certain malignancies (oral, laryngeal, uterine) and providing palliative benefit for others. Today, technological advances in high-energy radiation and diagnostic imaging have led to targeted intensity-modulated radiation therapy (IMRT) and have significantly reduced the risk of exposure for normal tissues.

1931—Colorado dentist Frederick McKay and others identify excess **fluoride** in local water supplies as the cause of dental mottling called "Colorado brown stain." The condition, now known as fluorosis, makes dental enamel unusually resistant to decay. By 1945 the U.S. Public Health Service (USPHS) recognizes the role of **fluoride** in preventing dental caries. The city of Grand Rapids, Michigan, becomes first in the world to fluoridate its drinking water. Follow-up studies show that the rate of tooth decay in thousands of children drops by over 60%. Fluoridation, endorsed by the USPHS in 1950, is one of the most successful public health measures ever advocated.

1932—Gerhard Domagk develops the first **sulfa** drug from a red dye called prontosil. Its sulfonamide portion is effective against many severe streptococcal infections.

1932—Albert Hyman invents an artificial **cardiac pacemaker**, which supplies an adjustable voltage current to restart the heart after arrest.

1932–1935—Max Theiler at the Rockefeller Institute develops a **vaccine against yellow fever**, an acute viral disease spread by infected mosquitoes.

1933—The development of high-resolution **electron microscopy** is a scientific breakthrough. In the field of virology it makes possible the detection and characterization of viruses and their interaction with infected cells.

1933—William Kouwenhoven's research on the cardiac effects of electric shock leads to the development of the **cardiac defibrillator** and **cardiopulmonary resuscitation**, or **CPR**.

1935—Edward Kendall and Tadeus Reichstein independently isolate **cortisone**, a hormone produced by the adrenal gland. Cortisone becomes the foremost drug in the treatment of inflammatory disease.

1936—**Hard (inflexible) plastic contact lenses** are introduced and replace glass lenses.

1937—Bernard Fantus establishes the first hospital "**blood bank**" at Cook County Hospital in Chicago, where his laboratory preserves and stores donor blood.

1937–1941—Daniel Bovet synthesizes the first **antihistamines** active against H1 receptors.

1938—Neuropsychiatrists Ugo Cerletti and Lucio Bini first administer **electroconvulsive therapy (ECT)** to a human patient. ECT is the only physical psychiatric therapy still in use; it is effective for the treatment of major depression.

1938–1941—Howard Florey and Ernst Chain succeed in producing the active component of Fleming's mold, **penicillin**. By the end of World War II penicillin has saved thousands from succumbing to life-threatening infections.

1940—Alexander Wiener and Philip Levine, together with Karl Landsteiner, identify the hereditary **Rh factor**, the cause of the feared hemolytic disease of the newborn. Their discovery leads to the development of Rh immune globulin prophylaxis for mothers.

1940—Charles Drew organizes collection and mass production of **dried blood plasma** as part of the "Blood for Britain" program to aid British soldiers and civilians during World War II. His blood storage techniques are instrumental in developing blood bank systems worldwide.

1940—Following an outbreak of an unusual bleeding disease in cattle, Karl Link and his students at the University of Wisconsin isolate an anticoagulant substance from spoiled sweet clover and name it dicoumarol, a fermentation product of the natural plant substance coumarin. In 1948, they develop a synthetic derivative, **warfarin** (from the acronym WARF, Wisconsin Alumni Research Foundation); it is initially used as a rat poison. **Warfarin (Coumadin)** is approved in 1954 for prevention and treatment of venous thrombosis (blood clots) and for thromboembolic complications of atrial fibrillation, cardiac valve replacement, heart attack, and stroke. It remains standard for long-term anticoagulant therapy.

1941—André Cournand and Dickinson Richards report on their **cardiac catheterization** studies, which help define cardiac physiology and pathophysiology of circulatory shock.

1941—George Papanicolaou and Herbert Traut publish the results of vaginal cell samplings in gynecological patients. Their findings establish the importance of the **Pap smear** in cervical cancer detection.

1942–1946—Alfred Gilman and Louis Goodman achieve temporary remission in lymphoma patients with infusion of nitrogen mustard, stimulating widespread research into **cancer chemotherapy**.

1943—Albert Schatz and Selman Waksman discover **streptomycin**, the first antibiotic effective for treating tuberculosis.

1943—Willem J. Kolff builds an "artificial kidney" during the Nazi occupation of Holland, using sausage casings, juice cans, and laundry tubs. In 1945 he carries out the first successful human **dialysis** with his apparatus, saving the life of a patient with renal failure.

1944—John Rock achieves successful **in vitro fertilization** of human eggs.

1947—American surgeon Claude Beck successfully reestablishes normal heart rhythm in a patient with ventricular fibrillation by applying the paddles of his defibrillator directly to the heart in the open chest. Beck's technique inspires the development of modern **cardiac defibrillators**.

1948—Optical technician Kevin Touhy accidentally creates a smaller **corneal contact lens** while sanding down a traditional full scleral lens. It proves a major improvement and remains the type of lens used today.

1948—Microbiologist John Enders succeeds in culturing **poliovirus**.

1948—Sidney Farber's research on folate antagonists leads to the first use of **methotrexate** in childhood leukemia.

1949—Harold Ridley successfully implants an **artificial intraocular lens** made of lightweight Plexiglas after removing a cataract.

1949—Anesthesiologist Virginia Apgar devises a system for rapid assessment of newborn infants. Known as the **Apgar Score**, it scores criteria such as **A**ppearance (color), **P**ulse, **G**rimace (reflexes), **A**ctivity (tone), and **R**espiration.

1949—Radiologist Douglas Howry builds the first **ultrasound** machine. His device eventually evolves into B-mode (brightness mode) imaging.

1950—Richard Doll and Austin Bradford Hill publish the results of their groundbreaking **epidemiological studies linking smoking to cancer** of the lung.

1951—Carl Djerassi synthesizes norethindrone, the first **oral contraceptive**.

1951—John Reid and John Wild invent a **handheld ultrasound** device to detect breast cancer and other tumors.

1952—Paul Zoll develops the first **external cardiac pacemaker**. The device generates a pulse with two electrodes placed on the patient's bare chest but requires connection to an electrical outlet.

1952—French researchers discover the antipsychotic and sedative effects of **chlorpromazine (Thorazine)**. The drug's therapeutic success brings about radical changes in the treatment of psychosis worldwide and marks a turning point in psychiatric practice.

1953—Jonas Salk reports positive test results with his killed, inactivated **polio vaccine**. A large-scale trial leads to nationwide vaccination programs in 1955.

1953—Rosalind Franklin's and Maurice Wilkins's X-ray crystallography studies aid Francis Crick and James Watson in delineating the molecular **structure of DNA**, the chromosomal building blocks that store the genetic code of every living organism.

1953—John Gibbon performs the first successful open-heart operation with the **heart-lung bypass machine** he invented to support the patient's heart and lung functions intra-operatively. Cardiopulmonary bypass ushers in a new era in cardiac surgery.

1953—Sven-Ivar Seldinger develops a percutaneous technique using a sheath and a guidewire for introducing catheters in **cardiac catheterization** procedures. The Seldinger technique becomes standard for placement of central venous catheters and chest tubes and for many other percutaneous interventions.

1953—Inge Edler and Hellmuth Hertz succeed in producing **ultrasound** images of cardiac structures, including the first mitral valve **echocardiogram**. Their technique uses **Doppler ultrasound**, which measures blood flow and is named for Swedish physicist Christian Doppler.

1954—Joseph Murray and David Hume perform the first successful and permanent kidney transplant from a 24-year-old donor to his identical twin brother, proving that **human organ transplants** can be viable.

1955–1958—Live attenuated **oral polio vaccine** developed by Albert Sabin is successfully tried on millions of people in Mexico, Eastern Europe, Asia, and the Netherlands. It supersedes the Salk vaccine but is not licensed in the United States until 1961.

1957—Earl Bakken and C. Walton Lillehei develop the first portable **battery-powered external pacemaker**.

1957—Two new classes of psychopharmacologic agents are introduced for treating depression and anxiety disorders: the **tricyclic antidepressants** and the **MAOIs (monoamine oxidase inhibitors)**.

1958—Rune Elmqvist and Åke Senning in Sweden build the first fully **implantable pacemaker**.

1958—Edward Hon uses a handheld **ultrasound** transducer to detect fetal heartbeat. It is the first use of the **Doppler monitor** in prenatal diagnosis.

1958—Pennsylvania optometrist Robert Morrison uses hydrogel, a pliable and permeable new plastic developed by Czechoslovakian Otto Wichterle, to make the first **soft contact lenses**. They quickly supersede previous glass or hard acrylic models.

1958–1960s—Scientists discover the existence of **human leukocyte antigens (HLAs)**, highly specific and genetically determined substances that regulate immunological reactions. In transplants, "foreign" HLAs lead to graft rejection and graft vs. host disease. Tissue typing and HLA donor–recipient crossmatching are major breakthroughs in the 1980s and contribute to the development of **transplant medicine**.

1960s—Morris Collen creates a computerized record tracking patients' screenings and test results at Kaiser Permanente in California. His work stimulates further research and leads to development of **electronic medical record (EMR)** systems.

1960—William Kouwenhoven and Jim Jude report on the benefits of rhythmic closed-chest compressions in cardiac arrest and lay the foundation for modern **cardiopulmonary resuscitation (CPR)**.

1960—The U.S. Food and Drug Administration (FDA) approves a combined estrogen-progesterone drug for use as **oral contraceptive**.

1960—Leo Sternbach develops the **benzodiazepine** Librium, the first in a highly effective class of anti-anxiety drugs. It is followed three years later by Valium, which becomes one of the most successful prescription drugs in history.

1960—Surgeon Albert Starr and engineer Lowell Edwards design a **mechanical heart valve**, which they successfully implant in the mitral position. Since then, technological advances in prostheses have extended the lives of thousands of patients with valvular disease.

1961—Ernest McCulloch and James Till prove the existence of blood-forming **stem cells** in the bone marrow. Their research explains why healthy bone marrow transplants can replace diseased or destroyed bone marrow.

1962—John Charnley pioneers a low-friction **artificial hip replacement** procedure using a polyethylene-stainless steel prosthesis. His design principles are applied in developing metal and plastic replacement devices for other diseased joints.

1963—Vascular radiologist Charles Dotter accidentally carries out the first successful **angioplasty**.

1963—Ian Donald uses **ultrasound** to detect early stages of gestation. Today ultrasonography is standard in prenatal diagnosis.

1963—**Combination chemotherapy** is shown to be superior to single agents in the treatment of some types of hematologic cancers.

1963–1970—American scientists John Enders and Maurice Hilleman develop the **measles, mumps, and rubella vaccines**. In 1971 a triple combination vaccine containing live attenuated measles, mumps, and rubella (MMR) virus is licensed for use. Since then, the incidence of these common childhood infections has been dramatically reduced worldwide. In the case of rubella, systematic vaccination has eliminated both congenital and acquired infections from a number of developed countries.

1964—**Laser photocoagulation** is introduced to treat diabetic retinopathy, a leading cause of blindness.

1965—Frank Pantridge installs the first **portable defibrillator** in a Belfast ambulance, effectively creating the first mobile coronary care unit. The apparatus weighs 110 pounds and is powered by car batteries.

1967—Cleveland Clinic surgeon René Favaloro performs one of the first successful **coronary artery bypass graft (CABG)** procedures, restoring coronary flow using the patient's own saphenous vein. Saphenous vein grafting is the most common CABG technique until the mid-1980s when studies show improved outcomes with internal thoracic and other arterial grafts. CABG is the most common cardiac operation; in 2010, a total of 395,000 procedures are recorded in the United States.

1967—Ophthalmologist Charles Kelman introduces ultrasonic **phacoemulsification** of the opacified lens to replace extracapsular extraction of cataracts.

1967—Sir Godfrey Hounsfield develops the first CT scanner, a major advance in diagnostic imaging. **Computer-assisted tomography (CT or CAT)** combines X-ray and computer technology to produce cross-sectional images of the body.

1967—South African surgeon Christiaan Barnard performs the first **human heart transplant** on a 53-year-old man; the patient died 18 days later.

1967—Baruch Blumberg isolates HBsAg, the surface antigen of the **hepatitis B virus** (HBV), also known as Australia antigen. His discovery leads to the development of the first hepatitis B vaccine.

1970—**Cyclosporine** is extracted from a Norwegian soil fungus. The compound selectively suppresses T-lymphocytes and is the first single agent to control organ rejection. It has been used in transplant patients since 1978.

1970–1973—American scientists Stanley Cohen, Herbert Boyer, and others develop **recombinant DNA** (rDNA) technology, which makes possible intracellular creation of artificial sequences of DNA nucleotides. Along with polymerase chain reaction (PCR), the method can replicate specific DNA sequences. It is used to identify and map genes and to analyze gene expression. Important medical applications include diagnostic tests for HIV infection and recombinant hepatitis B vaccine. Recombinant human insulin, the first drug developed with rDNA technology, was licensed in 1980 and today has almost completely replaced animal insulin.

1971–1973—Raymond Damadian, Paul Lauterbur, and Peter Mansfield develop **magnetic resonance imaging (MRI)**. MRI uses electromagnetic fields to manipulate atomic particles and analyze emitted radio signals in order to create a three-dimensional image. The technique has become key in diagnostic imaging of internal tissues and organs.

1972—Andreas Grüntzig pioneers the **balloon catheter** technique for **percutaneous angioplasty**.

1972—James Black demonstrates the existence of **H2 histamine receptors**, which mediate gastric acid secretion. His work leads to the development of the H2 antagonist cimetidine (Tagamet).

1975—Cesar Milstein and Georges Köhler produce the first **monoclonal antibodies (mAbs)**. Their technique makes possible the generation of unlimited supplies of highly specific immunoglobulins.

1975—The selective serotonin reuptake inhibitor (**SSRI) fluoxetine** is patented as a weight loss drug. In 1988 it is marketed as **Prozac** for the treatment of depression and obsessive-compulsive disorders.

1977—The first commercial full-body **PET (positron emission tomography)** scanner is introduced after Michael Phelps and others develop a PET camera in 1973. PET scanning studies metabolic activity through the regional tissue uptake of radioisotopes of a biological tracer molecule. In clinical medicine it is mainly used to detect spread of cancer.

1977—Andreas Grüntzig carries out the first **coronary angioplasty** in a 37-year-old man.

1977—Robert Edwards and Patrick Steptoe succeed in establishing a first human **IVF (in vitro fertilization)** pregnancy. The world's first "test-tube" baby is born in 1978.

1978—The work of Akira Endo leads to the isolation of a compound eventually named lovastatin, one of a family of drugs that inhibit cholesterol synthesis in the liver. **Statins** are shown to reduce low-density lipoprotein (LDL) ("bad") cholesterol and thereby prevent atherosclerotic cardiovascular disease.

1983—Françoise Barré-Sinoussi and Luc Montagnier discover the **human immunodeficiency virus (HIV),** a retrovirus that attacks the immune system and proves to be the cause of AIDS. Their discovery is crucial in targeting treatments for infected patients.

1983—Barry Marshall and J. Robin Warren report their findings that **Helicobacter pylori** is the likely cause of most peptic ulcers and gastritis. Their work revolutionizes the treatment of peptic ulcer disease.

1983—Kary Mullis develops the **polymerase chain reaction (PCR)**, a technique that replicates a particular DNA sequence and can generate, in a test tube, millions of copies of this DNA segment within a few hours. The PCR method has vast applications. In medical diagnostics it detects the presence of small amounts of foreign viral or bacterial DNA to diagnose infections. In genetic medicine, PCR can test for specific gene mutations that underlie hereditary disease. It is also used for tissue typing in transplant medicine, for sequencing and cloning of genes, and for detection of oncogenes, mutated genes that may induce growth of cancer cells.

1985—**Zidovudine (azidothymidine or AZT)**, an antiretroviral drug synthesized in 1964, is first tried on HIV-infected volunteers. The FDA grants accelerated approval for use against HIV and AIDS less than two years later. Since then, over 25 anti-HIV drugs have become available and are used in various combinations to decrease development of resistance. Modern HIV/AIDS therapies, especially HAART (highly active antiretroviral therapy) cocktails, have dramatically improved outcomes, turning a deadly infection into a chronic disease with good long-term survival.

1986—French cardiologist Jacques Puel implants the first **intravascular stent**, a wire mesh tube serving as an internal coronary scaffold, to prevent sudden closure and restenosis after transluminal coronary angioplasty. In 1987, a **balloon-expandable stent** invented by vascular radiologist Julio Palmaz is miniaturized for coronary use and implanted. It is used successfully in most percutaneous coronary angioplasties in the 1990s. Since 2002, the advent of **drug-eluting stents** reduces the rate of vascular restenosis even further. These drug-coated stents slowly release an antiproliferative agent to block fibrosis and scarring.

1986—A genetically engineered, **recombinant DNA hepatitis B vaccine** is approved 20 years after discovery of the virus, replacing earlier inactivated vaccines derived from plasma of HBV-positive donors. Infants are now routinely vaccinated against hepatitis B in many countries, which has led to a marked reduction in liver infections and liver cancer.

1987–1988—Harvey Alter and Michael Houghton succeed in identifying the **hepatitis C** virus, a major cause of infectious hepatitis throughout the world. Their discovery is a key factor in eliminating post-transfusion hepatitis.

1988—New York ophthalmologist Steven Trokel uses a computerized excimer laser to perform the first human corneal refractive surgery. By 2010, **laser vision correction (LASIK)** has been successfully performed in millions of patients worldwide.

1991–1993—Australian and U.S. immunologists develop the first human papilloma virus (**HPV) vaccines**. In 2006 the U.S. FDA approves Gardasil and Cervarix to protect against cancers due to persistent infection with certain viral strains.

1998–2006—American biologist James Thomson successfully isolates and cultures **human embryonic stem cells**. In 2006, Shinya Yamanaka in Japan pioneers a method to convert specialized adult cells into pluripotent "**induced" stem cells (iPSC)**. The discovery that "mature cells can be reprogrammed to become pluripotent" holds great potential for many avenues of research, including drug development and cellular pathophysiology in disease. In the field of regenerative medicine, iPSCs obviate the need for embryonic stem cells, since they, too, can give rise to specialized cell types and be used to repair or replace specific damaged or diseased tissues.

2000–2003—The international collaborative **Human Genome Project (HPG)** is drafted and completed. Initiated in 1990, the HPG identifies and maps the DNA sequences of 3 billion chemical base pairs that make up roughly 20,000 human genes. One of the most important investigations undertaken in modern medical science, it has numerous medical applications, including targeted drug design and identification of genes associated with hereditary forms of cancer.

Glossary

Acetabulum—cupped, concave socket on the side of each hip (pelvic) bone, which houses the ball-shaped head of the femur

Afferent—conducting or conveying toward the interior or the center (Latin *ad-* and *ferre*, to bring to); used to indicate direction (of flow) in blood vessels or nerve conduction; opposite of **efferent**

Agglutination—the sticking or clumping together to form a mass

Allograft—tissue graft from a donor of the same species, but who is not genetically identical to the recipient

Analgesic—pain reliever, or relieving pain (adj. or noun)

Anaphylaxis—acute, potentially life-threatening reaction to an antigenic substance, to which the body is hypersensitive

Anastomosis—surgical connection between blood vessels or other adjacent body parts

Angiography—imaging, usually by X-ray, of blood vessels after injection of radio-opaque contrast dye

Angioplasty—surgical procedure to dilate and remodel a narrowed or occluded artery by introducing and inflating a thin tube, or catheter, so as to improve blood flow

Antiscorbutic—agent that prevents or fights scurvy, a disease resulting from vitamin C deficiency (French, *scorbut*)

Armamentarium—medications, techniques, and materials available to medical practitioners (Latin for arsenal, weaponry)

Arthroplasty—surgical remodeling or replacement of a joint

Arrhythmia—abnormal or irregular rhythm or heartbeat

Atrium—one of the two upper chambers of the heart (in Roman architecture, the open central space or entrance court of a dwelling)

Auscultation—the listening for sounds within the body with the ear, but more usually with a stethoscope, to aid in diagnosis

Autograft—tissue graft transferred from one part of the body to another in the same individual

Bacteriostatic—capable of slowing or inhibiting bacterial growth and proliferation; compare to **bactericidal**, capable of killing bacteria

Blastocyst—mammalian embryo at a very early stage

Cardioplegia—technique used in cardiac surgery to arrest the heart artificially by injecting a salt solution, by inducing hypothermia, or by electrical stimulation

Cardiotomy—surgical incision into the heart

Cardioversion—medical procedure using electric current or medication to convert an abnormal heart rate or rhythm and restore it to normal function

Cholecystectomy—surgical extraction of the gallbladder

Cirrhosis—degenerative liver disease due to chronic inflammation, leading to excess fiber deposition and scarring of functional tissue

Clone—cell or organism with a genetic makeup identical to one or more others and derived from a common parent by asexual reproduction or created artificially; also DNA segment reproduced by genetic engineering

Craniostomy—surgical opening of the skull

Cystoscope—instrument inserted into the urethra for examining the urinary bladder

Cytoplasm—substance, or protoplasm, of a living cell, which surrounds its nucleus and is enclosed by the cytoplasmic membrane

Cytotoxic—poisonous or destructive to living cells

Decoction—concentrated liquid resulting from heating or boiling down a substance so as to extract its essence; often used for medicinal substances prepared from plant materials, such as leaves, roots, stems, or bark.

Diffraction—displacement and spreading out of a beam of light or a wave of sound or water as a result of encountering an obstacle or passing through a narrow opening

DNA (deoxyribonucleic acid)—double-helix molecule consisting of two strands of sugar and phosphate groups attached to one of four bases—adenine, thymine, guanine, or cytosine. DNA is the substance of the **chromosomes** located in the nucleus of all cells and carries the **genes**, each of which is a segment of a DNA molecule.

Egophony—change in vocal resonance in auscultation of the chest

Embolism—blocking of a blood vessel by an obstructing embolus, usually a clot of blood, a fat particle, or an air bubble

Embolus (emboli)—loose intravascular solid or gaseous particle carried by the bloodstream from its point of origin to a remote site where it lodges to cause an embolism

Encephalopathy—disease affecting the function of the brain

Endocardial—relating to the endocardium, the membrane that lines the inside of the heart

Endoscopy—procedure in which a flexible fiber-optic instrument is introduced into the body to inspect internal tissues (from the Greek *endo*, within, and *skopein*, to view)

Epilepsy—central nervous system disease characterized by sudden episodes of convulsions, loss of consciousness, or other sensorimotor disturbances and associated with abnormal electrical activity of the brain; seizure disorder

Erythrocyte—blood cell containing hemoglobin, the pigment that gives blood a red color, and that transports oxygen and carbon dioxide; red blood cell

Exfoliative—flaking off or shedding

Formalin—water solution of formaldehyde used as a preservative for scientific specimens

Galvanometer—instrument invented by Luigi Galvani to detect and measure small electric currents

Gene—basic functional unit of heredity, consisting of a distinct segment of chromosomal DNA, which determines and encodes hereditary traits and characteristics; each gene codes for a specific protein

Genome—total genetic material of an organism comprising all DNA contained in its chromosomes; the human genome is made up of 23 pairs of chromosomes

Genotype—genetic makeup of an individual organism or a cell

Glycosuria—excretion of glucose into the urine, nearly always due to untreated or undertreated diabetes

HeLa **cells**—first immortal human cell line maintained in tissue culture since February 1951, derived from cervical cancer tissue biopsied from a 31-year-old Baltimore patient named Henrietta Lacks. The (unwitting) patient died the same year. HeLa cells are used in medical research all over the world.

Hematopoiesis—production of blood cells by growth and differentiation of pluripotential stem cells in the bone marrow

Hemoglobinuria—presence or excretion of free hemoglobin in the urine; see also hematuria, glycosuria, etc.

Hemolysis—breakdown or destruction of red blood cells; can result from certain infections, poisons, or severe allergic reactions

Hepatocellular—pertaining to liver cells (hepatocytes)

Holter monitor—portable device for continuous recording of the electrical activity of the heart with chest electrodes, usually for 24 hours; named for biophysicist Norman Holter

Homocystinuria—hereditary disease due to an enzyme deficiency, which leads to an excess of homocysteine in the blood and the presence of its oxidized form in the urine

Hybridoma—hybrid cell line produced by the fusion of a myeloma tumor cell with an antibody-producing B-lymphocyte; the resulting hybridoma can produce large amounts of normal antibody, termed "monoclonal"

Immunoglobulin—protein molecule in the blood plasma secreted by B-lymphocytes and acting as antibody against a specific antigen in the body's immune response

Insufflation—blowing of gas, air, or aerosolized powdered medication into the lungs or other body cavity

Intracytoplasmic—within the cytoplasm

In vitro—performed or occurring in a laboratory test tube or culture dish; from the Latin, "in glass"

In vivo—occurring within a living organism

Laparoscopy—surgical procedure allowing visual examination of internal abdominal structures and organs by means of a laparoscope, a fiber-optic instrument inserted through a small incision in the abdominal wall, after insufflating carbon dioxide into the abdominal cavity; from the Greek, *lapara,* flank

Lysis—destruction, dissolution, disintegration

Miasma—noxious odor or atmosphere; in ancient medicine, it was held that certain diseases were caused by the presence of poisonous vapors, or miasma, in the air; from the Greek *miasma*, pollution

Mesenchyme (mesenchymal)—undifferentiated embryonic connective tissue that gives rise to connective and skeletal tissues, including blood and lymph vessels

Monaural—involving the use of one ear; compare to binaural

Monoclonal—pertaining to, or derived from, a single clone, usually of cells; monoclonal antibodies (mAb) are specific antibodies made by identical immune cells, all cloned of a unique parent cell; compare to polyclonal (made from several different clones)

Myxedema—condition characterized by dry coarse skin, hair loss, weight gain, mental slowing, and cold intolerance, typically associated with hypothyroidism

Nucleotide—organic compound forming the structural unit of DNA, consisting of a purine or pyrimidine base linked to a sugar and phosphate group

Osteogenic—involved in bone formation

Pancreatectomy—surgical removal or extraction of the pancreas

Pathogenic—causing or capable of causing disease

Peptic—relating to pepsin, the main digestive enzyme in the stomach that breaks down proteins; relating to digestion

Perfusion—flow or supply of fluid, especially blood, to tissues or organs by circulating it through blood vessels

Pectoriloquy—characteristic transmission of the patient's voice sounds through the chest wall during auscultation

Phagocytic—pertaining to phagocytes; a phagocyte is a specialized cell capable of engulfing and digesting bacteria, cell and cell debris, and other particles; see also phagocytosis

Phenylketonuria—inherited enzymatic deficiency rendering the patient unable to metabolize the essential amino acid phenylalanine

Pluripotential—capable of giving rise to various different cell types; also pluripotent

Pneumoencephalography—radiographic technique formerly used in the X-ray diagnosis of intracranial disease by introducing air into the ventricles of the brain in order to displace the cerebrospinal fluid and act as a contrast medium

Pneumothorax—presence of air in the pleural cavity causing the lung to collapse; it can be spontaneous or due to injury of the lung or the chest wall

Pneumoperitoneum—presence of air or gas in the peritoneal cavity, usually due to perforation of the intestinal tract; it is artificially induced in diagnostic laparoscopy

Polypectomy—surgical removal of a polyp

Prosthesis—artificial device used as replacement for a body part or to correct an abnormality

Puerperal—relating to childbirth or the period immediately following it, usually about six weeks; see also puerperium; from Latin *puer*, child

Râle—abnormal rattling sound heard in pulmonary auscultation; from the French, *râle*

Randomization—process of making random; often applied to random assignment of participants or use of treatments in experimental design

Retinitis pigmentosa—hereditary eye disease characterized by progressive loss of vision

Revisionism—theory or practice of modifying accepted interpretations in politics or history

Rhonchus (pl. **rhonchi**)—abnormal sound produced by air passing through narrowed bronchi, heard during auscultation; often described as musical or snoring

Sepsis—infectious condition in which disease-causing microbes or toxins destroy soft tissues and/or invade the bloodstream

Sigmoidoscopy—examination of the rectum and sigmoid colon by means of a rigid or flexible tube inserted through the anus; see also colonoscopy

Sonography—producing a graphic representation with the use and analysis of sound waves to assess the presence of solids in a fluid medium

Speculum—instrument inserted into the opening of a cavity such as the vagina or nasal orifice and dilating it for the purpose of inspection

Sphygmomanometer—instrument for measuring blood pressure

Stenosis—narrowing or constriction of a duct or an opening, such as a blood vessel or heart valve

Tamponade (cardiac)—compression of the heart, a dangerous condition resulting from accumulation of fluid around the heart muscle within the non-distensible pericardial sac

Teleological—relating to a goal, aim, or result; pertaining to teleology, the explanation of natural phenomena by means of a purpose or utility they serve

Toxin—poison or poisonous substance produced by an animal, plant, or microorganism

Toxoid—poisonous substance that has been rendered harmless, usually by chemical treatment, so as to reduce its toxicity while retaining its antigenic property; used in vaccines

Toxigenic—producing toxin or toxic effects

Transluminal—passing or passed through a passage or opening; from the Latin, *trans-*, across, and *lumen*, light

Trendelenburg—proper name, after German surgeon Friedrich Trendelenburg; he devised a number of techniques and tests named for him

Tomography—diagnostic imaging technique by which thin sections or slices of a three-dimensional image of a body part or of internal organs are reproduced

Trocar—instrument with a sharp, three-cornered point and a cannula to withdraw fluids from internal body cavities and spaces

Ventroscopy—examination of the abdominal cavity by means of an instrument; see also laparoscopy; from the Latin, *venter*, stomach, belly

Virulence—relative severity or intensity of a disease or poison; disease-producing capacity of a microbe

Index

About the Author

CHRISTIANE NOCKELS FABBRI, PhD, a native of Luxembourg, has practiced clinical medicine since 1984, most recently at Yale Health in New Haven, Connecticut. She studied psychology at Aix-en-Provence and medicine at Strasbourg and was certified in physician associate studies by the Yale School of Medicine, where she later served as the PA Program associate director. She holds a master of philosophy degree in medieval studies and a doctorate in the history of medicine from Yale University, where her research focused on medieval and early modern plague. Her published works include an essay on the therapeutic value of theriac as an early plague remedy ("Treating Medieval Plague" in *Early Science and Medicine*) and an edited translation of "Angelo Mosso's Circulation of Blood in the Human Brain."